Breast Disorders

Editors

VICTORIA L. GREEN
PATRICE M. WEISS

OBSTETRICS AND GYNECOLOGY CLINICS OF NORTH AMERICA

www.obgyn.theclinics.com

Consulting Editor
WILLIAM F. RAYBURN

September 2013 • Volume 40 • Number 3

ELSEVIER

1600 John F. Kennedy Boulevard • Suite 1800 • Philadelphia, Pennsylvania, 19103-2899

http://www.theclinics.com

OBSTETRICS AND GYNECOLOGY CLINICS OF NORTH AMERICA Volume 40, Number 3
September 2013 ISSN 0889-8545, ISBN-13: 978-0-323-18864-7

Editor: Kerry Holland

Obstetrics and Gynecology Clinics (ISSN 0889-8545) is published quarterly by Elsevier Inc., 360 Park Avenue South, New York, NY 10010-1710. Months of issue are March, June, September, and December. Periodicals postage paid at New York, NY, and additional mailing offices. Subscription price per year is $293.00 (US individuals), $518.00 (US institutions), $146.00 (US students), $353.00 (Canadian individuals), $652.00 (Canadian institutions), $214.00 (Canadian students), $428.00 (foreign individuals), $652.00 (foreign institutions), and $214.00 (foreign students). To receive student/resident rate, orders must be accompanied by name of affiliated institution, date of term, and the signature of program/residency coordinator on institution letterhead. Orders will be billed at individual rate until proof of status is received. Foreign air speed delivery is included in all *Clinics* subscription prices. All prices are subject to change without notice. POSTMASTER: Send address changes to *Obstetrics and Gynecology Clinics*, Elsevier Health Sciences Division, Subscription Customer Service, 3251 Riverport Lane, Maryland Heights, MO 63043. **Customer Service: Telephone: 1-800-654-2452 (U.S. and Canada); 314-447-8871 (outside U.S. and Canada). Fax: 314-447-8029. E-mail: journalscustomerservice-usa@elsevier.com (for print support); journalsonlinesupport-usa@elsevier.com (for online support).**

Reprints. For copies of 100 or more of articles in this publication, please contact the Commercial Reprints Department, Elsevier Inc., 360 Park Avenue South, New York, New York 10010-1710. Tel.: 212-633-3874; Fax: 212-633-3820; E-mail: reprints@elsevier.com.

Obstetrics and Gynecology Clinics of North America is also published in Spanish by McGraw-Hill Interamericana Editores S.A., P.O. Box 5-237, 06500, Mexico; in Portuguese by Reichmann and Affonso Editores, Rio de Janeiro, Brazil; and in Greek by Paschalidis Medical Publications, Athens, Greece.

Obstetrics and Gynecology Clinics of North America is covered in MEDLINE/PubMed (Index Medicus), Excerpta Medica, Current Concepts/Clinical Medicine, Science Citation Index, BIOSIS, CINAHL, and ISI/BIOMED.

Printed and bound by CPI Group (UK) Ltd, Croydon, CR0 4YY

Transferred to digital print 2012

Contributors

CONSULTING EDITOR

WILLIAM F. RAYBURN, MD, MBA
Randolph V. Seligman Endowed Professor and Chair, Department of Obstetrics and Gynecology, University of New Mexico School of Medicine, Albuquerque, New Mexico

EDITORS

VICTORIA L. GREEN, MD, JD, MBA
Associate Professor, Department of Gynecology and Obstetrics; Director, Gynecology Breast Clinic, Avon Comprehensive Breast Center, Winship Cancer Institute, Emory University School of Medicine, Emory University, Atlanta, Georgia

PATRICE M. WEISS, MD
Chair and Professor, Department of Obstetrics and Gynecology, Virginia Tech Carilion School of Medicine and Research Institute, Carilion Clinic, Roanoke, Virginia

AUTHORS

LISA ATKINSON, RTR(M), BS
Manager, Breast Care Center, Carilion Roanoke Community Hospital, Roanoke, Virginia

CECELIA A. BELLCROSS, PhD, MS
Assistant Professor of Human Genetics, Director, Genetic Counselor Training Program, Emory University School of Medicine, Atlanta, Georgia

BEVERLY H. BINNER, JD
Carilion Clinic Legal Department, Carilion Clinic, Roanoke, Virginia

OTIS W. BRAWLEY, MD, FACP, FASCO
American Cancer Society, Emory University, Atlanta, Georgia

EMILY GANNON, BS
Department of Radiology, Carilion Clinic, Roanoke, Virginia

EVELYN M. GARCIA, MD
Chairman and Medical Director, Department of Radiology, Carilion Clinic; Assistant Professor of Radiology, Virginia Tech Carilion School of Medicine, Roanoke, Virginia

VICTORIA L. GREEN, MD, JD, MBA
Associate Professor, Department of Gynecology and Obstetrics; Director, Gynecology Breast Clinic, Avon Comprehensive Breast Center, Winship Cancer Institute, Emory University at Grady Memorial Hospital, Emory University, Atlanta, Georgia

CATHERINE HAGAN-AYLOR, BA, BSN, MSN, CBCN
Carilion Clinic Breast Care Center, Department of Radiology, Carilion Clinic, Roanoke, Virginia

EILEEN KENNY, MD
Section Chief Breast Imaging, Breast Care Center, Carilion Roanoke Community Hospital; Assistant Professor of Radiology, Virginia Tech Carilion School of Medicine, Roanoke, Virginia

IRIS KRISHNA, MD, MPH
Department of Gynecology and Obstetrics, Division of Maternal-Fetal Medicine, Emory University School of Medicine, Atlanta, Georgia

MICHAEL LINDSAY, MD, MPH
Department of Gynecology and Obstetrics, Division of Maternal-Fetal Medicine, Emory University School of Medicine, Atlanta, Georgia

DANA MEANEY-DELMAN, MD, MPH
Adjunct Assistant Professor of Gynecology and Obstetrics, Emory University School of Medicine, Atlanta, Georgia

LISA S. MITCHELL, MBA
Regional Practice Director, Department of Radiology, Carilion Clinic, Roanoke, Virginia

JAMES MULLET, MD
Breast Imaging Radiologist, Carilion Clinic; Associate Professor of Radiology, Virginia Tech Carilion School of Medicine, Roanoke, Virginia

ANITA L. NELSON, MD
Professor, Department of Obstetrics and Gynecology, Harbor-UCLA Medical Center, Torrance, California

MICHAELA ONSTAD, MD, MPH
Breast Surgery Fellow, Program in Women's Oncology, Department of Obstetrics and Gynecology, Women and Infants Hospital, Warren Alpert Medical School of Brown University, Providence, Rhode Island

ERIK S. STORM, DO
Breast Care Center, Carilion Roanoke Community Hospital; Assistant Professor of Radiology, Virginia Tech Carilion School of Medicine, Roanoke, Virginia

ASHLEY STUCKEY, MD
Assistant Professor, Program in Women's Oncology, Department of Obstetrics and Gynecology, Women and Infants Hospital, Warren Alpert Medical School of Brown University, Providence, Rhode Island

PATRICE M. WEISS, MD
Chair and Professor, Department of Obstetrics and Gynecology, Virginia Tech Carilion School of Medicine and Research Institute, Carilion Clinic, Roanoke, Virginia

AMELIA B. ZELNAK, MD, MSc
Assistant Professor of Hematology and Medical Oncology, Winship Cancer Institute, Emory University School of Medicine, Atlanta, Georgia

Contents

> The number of women diagnosed with breast cancer continues to
> increase, but mortality rates have substantially declined. Much of the
> credit for this decline has been attributed to early detection from mammo-
> graphic screening. However, there are significant controversies about
> the effectiveness of all screening tools for breast cancer, concerns about
> the potential harm that can result from screening, and questions about the
> appropriateness of screening recommendations. One of the greatest bar-
> riers to achieving consensus is the lack of agreement about the purpose of
> screening efforts. This article reviews many of the current controversies
> and attempts to clarify the arguments.

> Mammography will continue as the breast cancer screening imaging study
> of choice for the foreseeable future. Ultrasound and magnetic resonance
> imaging (MRI) are widely available adjunctive studies for women with sus-
> picious mammographic or clinical findings, and MRI is a screening tool for
> women with specific increased risks for breast cancer. Options for diagno-
> sis will continue to evolve and progress. This article discusses a wide
> variety of imaging options currently used and in development, their
> strengths, limitations, and potential future roles in the continuing pursuit
> of early breast cancer diagnosis, treatment, and follow-up.

> Full understanding of benign breast disease should enable the obs-
> tetrician-gynecologist to appropriately evaluate symptoms, distinguish
> between benign and malignant processes, determine which benign breast
> lesions require surgical management, and identify patients who are at
> increased risk of developing breast cancer. This article reviews nipple dis-
> charge, breast pain, palpable breast masses, adolescent breast disorders,
> inflammatory lesions (including mastitis and breast abscesses), and benign
> breast abnormality detected on imaging and biopsy. Each topic provides
> a review of the clinical presentation, a discussion of the appropriate
> workup, and a further description of specific etiology within each category.

An understanding of the diagnosis and clinical management of hereditary
breast and ovarian cancer syndrome (HBOC) is essential for obstetricians/
gynecologists. This article provides practical information regarding collecting a family history, cancer risk assessment and genetic testing,
BRCA-associated cancer prognosis and treatment, screening recommendations, and prevention strategies. Through appropriate cancer risk
assessment, women with BRCA1/2 mutations can be identified, and
screening and prevention strategies can be used before a diagnosis of
cancer occurs. Women's health providers with a strong working knowledge of HBOC are able to improve the quality of care for women and families impacted by BRCA1/2 mutations.

There has been a growing Black-White disparity in breast cancer mortality
after a period of relative equivalence. Literature shows that Black Americans with breast cancer are less likely to receive optimal care compared
with White Americans. Tumors in Black Americans are more likely to be
poorly differentiated and estrogen receptor negative and exhibit a high
S-phase fraction compared with tumors from White Americans. Differences in dietary habits, breast-feeding, and obesity account for some of
the population differences in outcome among Black Americans.

Today breast cancer remains a major public health problem, although
reducing its risk is now an achievable medical objective. Risk-assessment
models may be used in estimating a woman's risk for developing breast
cancer and to direct suitable candidates for preventive therapy. Researchers
are attempting to enhance individualized risk assessment through incorporation of phenotypic biomarkers. Individual selective estrogen receptor
modulators have been approved for breast cancer risk reduction, and other
drug categories are being studied. It is critical that obstetrician-gynecologists
be familiar with the evolving science of the risk assessment of breast cancer
as well as interventional and surveillance strategies.

Most obstetrics and gynecology (OB/GYN) physicians assist their patients
at the time of a new breast cancer diagnosis. OB/GYN physicians can
assure women that the tests being performed to map the individual features of the breast cancer follow a predictable and organized process. In
many cases, it is appropriate to confidently reassure the patient of
a good outcome based on the diagnostic mammography features. Regular
attendance at interdisciplinary breast cancer conferences will help

OB/GYN physicians develop the required knowledge to counsel women with newly diagnosed breast cancer.

Iris Krishna and Michael Lindsay

Pregnancy-associated breast cancer is defined as breast cancer diagnosed during pregnancy or in the first postpartum year. Breast cancer is one of the more common malignancies to occur during pregnancy and, as more women delay childbearing, the incidence of breast cancer in pregnancy is expected to increase. This article provides an overview of diagnosis, staging, and treatment of pregnancy-associated breast cancer. Recommendations for management of breast cancer in pregnancy are discussed.

Amelia B. Zelnak

Long-term outcomes for early-stage breast cancer have continued to improve, and more patients are becoming long-term survivors. In addition to patients' concern about risk of developing recurrent disease, they are also concerned about potential toxicities of treatment. Current guidelines for long-term follow-up are reviewed. Potential toxicities of tamoxifen and aromatase inhibitors are reviewed. Management of menopausal symptoms, cancer-related fatigue, and cognitive function is discussed.

Lisa S. Mitchell, Lisa Atkinson, Catherine Hagan-Aylor, Beverly H. Binner, Emily Gannon, Patrice M. Weiss, and Eileen Kenny

A common endeavor shared by physicians practicing in specialty fields of Radiology and Obstetrics and Gynecology is the comprehensive care and diagnosis of women with breast problems and breast disease. Because each specialty provides its respective clinical expertise in breast health, each also shares a concern, which is the high risk of litigation associated with a missed or delayed diagnosis of breast cancer. This shared concern is well documented for both specialties. Instead, it is argued that physicians are better prepared by engaging in the practice of evidence-based breast care in their respective specialties.

OBSTETRICS AND GYNECOLOGY CLINICS

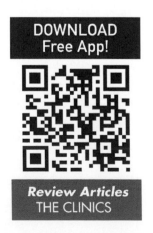

Foreword

Obstetrician-Gyenocologists are Primary Providers for Breast Health Maintenance and Education

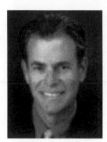

William F. Rayburn, MD, MBA
Consulting Editor

This issue of *Obstetrics and Gynecology of North America*, guest edited Dr Patrice M. Weiss and Dr Victoria L. Green, enlightens issues surrounding breast health and breast cancer. Obstetrician-gynecologists are the primary providers of breast health mainte-nance, breast education, and cancer screening and are now increasingly involved with diagnosis and management teams. Most women list breast cancer as one, if not their top, health concern. Similarly, ob-gyns struggle with the early diagnosis of this condi-tion, especially during pregnancy.

Breast cancer is the most common source of cancer in women and the second lead-ing cause of cancer death. Fortunately, annual mortality rates have decreased over the last decade. The authors discuss controversies surrounding mammography and other imaging modalities. Most but not all early breast cancers are diagnosed as a result of an abnormal screening mammogram.

Evaluation of the anxious woman with a breast problem requires a careful assessment of her presenting symptoms and physical findings on the breast and regional lymph node examination. It is important to evaluate complaints thoroughly to ensure that benign lesions and cancers are diagnosed and treated promptly, particularly because it is difficult to differentiate between fast- and slow-growing cancers. Continued support and careful communication remain essential, especially among those undergoing cancer treatment or who are survivors.

Most mammographic findings represent benign tissue. An abnormal screening mammogram usually requires additional evaluation with magnification views, spot compression views, and/or targeted ultrasonography to determine the need for tissue sampling. Ultrasound examination of the breast is an important diagnostic adjunct to

Obstet Gynecol Clin N Am 40 (2013) ix–x
http://dx.doi.org/10.1016/j.ogc.2013.08.002
0889-8545/13/$ – see front matter © 2013 Elsevier Inc. All rights reserved.

mammography to differentiate between solid and cystic masses and provide guidance for interventional procedures. Breast MRI is highly sensitive and can identify foci of cancer that are not evident on physical examination, mammogram, or ultrasound.

Many discrete palpable abnormalities are usually simple breast cysts and will need only confirmation with an ultrasound. A simple and asymptomatic cyst permits a trial of observation, while needle aspiration should be performed if the cysts are symptomatic or nonsimple. Masses that are solid on any imaging will require a biopsy to provide a histological diagnosis. Normal imaging should not be considered proof that malignancy is not present. The diagnostic procedure of choice for most solid masses is core needle biopsy rather than surgical biopsy.

Recent publications and news media stories have contributed to confusion regarding breast cancer screening. As it is often the ob-gyn providing breast health and education, the authors provide an overview about the hereditary breast and ovarian cancer syndrome to help guide providers on decisions of when and whom to screen. Hereditary breast and ovarian cancers are associated with mutations in two genes, breast cancer type 1 and 2 susceptibility genes (BRCA1 and BRCA2). Specific familial patterns and clinical features of hereditary breast and ovarian cancer, along with any accompanying other cancers, should be used to identify those individuals in need of genetic counseling, testing, and cancer surveillance.

On review of this issue, the reader should acquire more confidence to counsel patients, assess risk, screen with the appropriate modality, and offer preventive therapies. Contemporary management and treatment options are well described in this issue, and any suspicion of breast cancer requires that care be coordinated with several specialties. An integrated approach with breast imagers and breast surgeons can minimize unnecessary biopsies and expedite diagnosis for the woman who receives a diagnosis of breast cancer. I wish to thank the editors and authors for their timely attention to this important subject concerning all adult women.

William F. Rayburn, MD, MBA
Department of Obstetrics and Gynecology
University of New Mexico School of Medicine
MSC10 5580, 1 University of New Mexico
Albuquerque, NM 87131-0001, USA

E-mail address:
wrayburn@salud.unm.edu

Preface

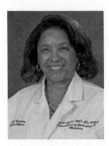 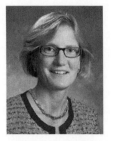

Victoria L. Green, MD, JD, MBA   Patrice M. Weiss, MD
Editors

Issues surrounding breast health and breast cancer have impacted most individuals personally, through a loved one, a friend, or a colleague. When reflecting on health and wellness, most women list breast cancer as one of, if not the top, concern. Moreover, breast cancer is the most common source of cancer in women and the second leading cause of cancer death. obstetrician-gynecologists have for long been the primary provider of breast health maintenance, breast education, and screening for women and are now increasingly involved in diagnosis, management, and cancer care. Recent publications and news media stories have contributed to confusion regarding breast cancer screening not only for patients but health care providers as well, thus prompting the need for a resource that provides the latest and most up-to-date knowledge in the field.

In this issue of *Obstetrics and Gynecology Clinics of North America*, we tap into the expertise of leaders in breast disorders. We seek to provide a multidisciplinary approach to breast disorders—recognizing that it is a team of health care providers from multiple specialties who care for women and breast disorders, especially breast cancer.

This issue begins with an immediate look at controversies regarding mammography, self breast exams, and clinical breast exams. As discussed, these areas lack universally accepted recommendations; thus, it was critical to clarify this concept first and to lay a foundation for subsequent articles.

Assisting the reader to understand the clinical significance of various breast modalities and their impact on breast care is addressed next; the author describes and explains the use, application, and limitations of each imaging modality.

As it is often the obstetrician-gynecologists providing breast health and education, we address both benign breast disorders and hereditary breast and ovarian cancer syndromes to help guide providers when and whom to screen.

One article is dedicated to delineation of Health Disparities and their impact on breast cancer and care. Their prevalence in breast cancer as well as other aspects of medicine is reviewed.

The widespread controversies existing for screening are also noted with breast cancer risk assessment and prevention. Next, an article written by a contributing

Obstet Gynecol Clin N Am 40 (2013) xi–xii
http://dx.doi.org/10.1016/j.ogc.2013.08.001
0889-8545/13/$ – see front matter © 2013 Published by Elsevier Inc.

radiologist emphasizes the role of the obstetrician-gynecologists in the breast health team.

Similarly, obstetrician-gynecologists struggle, as do patients, with the management and diagnosis of breast cancer in pregnancy. An article is dedicated to this topic and also addresses early stage breast cancer survivors.

Finally, out of respect and deference to the environment in which providers now practice, we conclude this issue with medical legal considerations in breast health and the need for collaboration between obstetrician-gynecologists and radiologists. This last article was written by a group of practitioners from a well-integrated and multispecialty breast care center where they discuss ideas to decrease the likelihood of litigation.

We hope you find this issue both educational and enlightening. We also hope you acquire additional skills and confidence to counsel patients as well as assess risk, screen with the appropriate modality, offer preventive therapies, and work collaboratively with other breast care health providers.

Victoria L. Green, MD, JD, MBA
Emory University School of Medicine
Department of Gynecology and Obstetrics
Glenn Building, 4th Floor
49 Jesse Hill Jr Drive
Atlanta, GA 30303, USA

Patrice M. Weiss, MD
Department of Obstetrics and Gynecology
Virginia Tech Carilion School of Medicine and Research Institute
2 Riverside Circle
Roanoke, VA 24016, USA

E-mail addresses:
vgree01@emory.edu (V.L. Green)
pmweiss@carolion.com (P.M. Weiss)

Controversies Regarding Mammography, Breast Self-Examination, and Clinical Breast Examination

Anita L. Nelson, MD

KEYWORDS

- Breast cancer screening • Breast self-examination • Clinical breast examination
- Mammography • Clinical guidelines

KEY POINTS

- The first step in a successful screening program is to identify women who are at a higher risk from those who fall into the general population risk category.
- In designing appropriate screening recommendations, the harms done by the screening test must be quantified and balanced against the benefits. The opportunity costs must also be factored in: what other services could be provided with the dollars used for intensively screening this disease?
- For the general population, routine breast self-examination is not useful, and frequent mammographic screening may cause more harm than benefits given the higher rates of false positivity.
- Women with a higher risk of developing breast cancer should be screened with more sensitive tests and more frequency. In addition to more intensive screening, interventions to reduce their risks should be strongly encouraged.

INTRODUCTION

Arguments about breast cancer screening recommendations have been in the public limelight for many years. Tensions have reached such high levels that, at times, politicians have convened congressional hearings. Guidelines from different professional organizations are inconsistent, differing not only in the tools to be used to detect early cancer but also in the age at which screening should begin and the frequency with which the tests should be performed (**Table 1**).[1,2] All 3 classic screening tests have

Disclosure Statement: The author has the following potential conflicts of interest: Bayer, Merck, Pfizer, Teva (grants/research); Bayer, Merck, Teva (honoraria/speakers bureau); Agile, Bayer, Ferring, Merck, Teva, Watson (consultant/advisory board).
Department of Obstetrics and Gynecology, Harbor-UCLA Medical Center, 1000 West Carson Street, Box 474, Torrance, CA 90509, USA
E-mail address: anitalnelson@earthlink.net

Obstet Gynecol Clin N Am 40 (2013) 413–427
http://dx.doi.org/10.1016/j.ogc.2013.05.001
0889-8545/13/$ – see front matter © 2013 Elsevier Inc. All rights reserved.

obgyn.theclinics.com

Table 1
Recommendations for breast cancer screening from various organizations

	Mammography	Clinical Breast Examination	Breast Self-Examination Instruction	Breast Self-Awareness
American College of Obstetricians and Gynecologists	Aged 40 y and older annually	Aged 20–39 y every 1–3 y Aged 40 y and older annually	Consider for high-risk patients	Recommended
American Cancer Society	Aged 40 y and older annually	Aged 20–39 y every 1–3 y Aged 40 y and older annually	Optional for those aged 20 y and older	Recommended
National Comprehensive Cancer Network	Aged 40 y and older annually	Aged 20–39 y every 1–3 y Aged 40 y and older annually	Recommended	Recommended
National Cancer Institute	Aged 40 y and older every 1–2 y	Recommended	Not recommended	—
US Preventative Services Task Force	Aged 50–74 y biennially	Insufficient evidence	Not recommended	—

Data from American College of Obstetricians-Gynecologists. Practice bulletin no. 122: breast cancer screening. Obstet Gynecol 2011;118:373.

come under scrutiny. Breast self-examination (BSE) is now considered to be optional or it is discouraged. The value of clinical breast examinations (CBE) is seen primarily in conjunction with imaging studies. Although credited by most authorities as having contributed to a decline in breast cancer mortality, mammography has been characterized by some as causing more harm than benefit. Conflicts in recommendations may leave clinicians at risk, especially if they follow more conservative guidelines. Such practice may also put clinicians at odds with their own patients. Often the decision of appropriate screening tools is left by default to third-party payers about which tests are covered by the patient's insurance.

The World Health Organization (WHO) recognizes that early detection remains the cornerstone of efforts to reduce breast cancer mortality.[3] In general, early detection of any disease can be achieved by either educating the at-risk population about early signs or symptoms or by screening the presumably asymptomatic population. Key to that success is an organized program targeting the right population.[4] The WHO has defined the properties needed for an appropriate screening test (**Box 1**).[5] According to those criteria, it is reasonable to invest in early breast cancer detection efforts. Breast cancer is an important health problem; the American Cancer Society estimates that in 2013, a total of 226,870 cases of breast cancer will be diagnosed in the United States and 39,510 women will die with their disease. Breast cancer risks increase progressively as women age, but there are important ethnic differences in both the absolute risks and their temporal patterns.[6] For Caucasian women, breast cancer risks start in their 20s and increase each year until 80 years of age. For African American women, breast cancer risks start in their teen years and progressively increase until 85 years of age, albeit at a lower absolute incidence than Caucasian women. Demographic shifts expected in the United States in the next 2 decades mean that groups

---

Box 1
WHO criteria for disease screening

- The condition that is screened for should represent a major cause of death and have a substantial prevalence in the population.

- The natural history of the disease, from latency to overt disease, should be well characterized.

- There should be a treatment of the disease's latent or early stage that improves the outcome.

- The screening test should be acceptable to the population.

- Effective treatments should be available for those with overt disease.

- Facilities for diagnosis and treatment should be available.

- There should be agreement among clinical guidelines on whom to treat.

- Screening should be cost-effective.

- Screening tests should have a high positive predictive value, negative predictive value, sensitivity, and specificity.

From Wilson JM, Jungner J. Principles and practice of screening for disease. World Health Organization; 1968; with permission.

---

with traditionally lower rates of breast cancer screening will experience significant increases in breast cancer. For example, by the year 2030, the total number of cases of breast cancer in the United States is expected to increase by 30%. However, in African American women, the numbers are projected to increase by 48%, those in Hispanic women are expected to increase 106%, and those in Asian/Pacific Island women will see a 100% increase.[7]

It is with better understanding of the natural history of breast cancer and better appreciation of the seen and unseen costs of the available screening tests that recommendations for screening have been reduced by some authorities. However, as witnessed by the variability seen in **Box 1**, those more modest screening standards are not accepted by many groups, especially by women themselves. Patient requests for early and frequent breast cancer screening tests are often based on the overestimation of the incidence of the disease, an inflated impression of the ability of screening tests to affect outcomes, and an under appreciation of the adverse impacts that those screening tests may themselves cause. Immediately following the announcement of the 2009 US Preventative Services Task Force's (USPSTF) recommendation that mammography screening start at 50 years of age, a *USA Today*/Gallop survey found that when asked to estimate a woman's risk of getting breast cancer in her 40s, 40% of respondents estimated that risk to be 20% to 50%. The real risk is 1.45% (**Table 2**).

Finally, conflicts among guidelines from different expert groups often result from fundamental differences in the outcome measures valued by those groups. For example, is the goal of screening to reduce breast cancer deaths or to maximize years of life gained? Is it necessary that benefits of screening greatly exceed the risks? Must the approach selected be the most cost-effective? This article explores each of these issues to help clarify the choices that need to be made when adopting breast cancer screening guidelines.

INDIVIDUALIZING SCREENING RECOMMENDATIONS

The first step in selecting appropriate breast cancer screening tests for any woman is to identify her personal risk factors for breast cancer. Important modifiable risk factors,

Table 2
Age-specific probabilities of developing invasive female breast cancer[a]

If Current Age Is...	The Probability of Developing Breast Cancer in the Next 10 y[b] (%)	Or 1 in
20	0.06	168
30	0.43	232
40	1.45	69
50	2.38	42
60	3.45	29
70	3.74	27
Lifetime risk	12.15	8

[a] Among those free of cancer at the beginning of the age interval. Based on cases diagnosed 2005 to 2007. Percentages and "1 in" numbers may not be numerically equivalent due to rounding.
[b] Probability derived using NCI DevCan Software, Version 6.5.0.
  Data from American Cancer Society. Breast cancer facts & figures 2009–2010. Atlanta (GA): American Cancer Society, Inc.

such as obesity[7,8] and excessive alcohol use,[9,10] should be discussed with women worried about breast cancer. Women without obviously high-risk family or personal histories should have their lifetime and 5-year risks of developing breast cancer quantified using one of the available breast cancer estimators. Unfortunately, as important as this first step is, only 18% of physicians reported using a computer algorithm to assess women's risks.[11] In another survey of primary care providers, 71% reported that they usually collected family history of breast cancer, but only a minority collected information about other important risk factors; more than three-quarters reported they never calculated a woman's risk, and half did not know what a Gail model was.[12] Clearly, all women are at risk of developing breast cancer, and risk factors other than family history are important.[13] Both the Gail model and the National Cancer Institute's Breast Cancer Assessment Tool are available at the following Web site: http://www.cancer.gov/bcrisktool/default.aspx. Calculating the probability a woman will develop detectable breast cancer in her lifetime often has significant value to her because that calculated estimate is generally much lower than she anticipates and can provide her the opportunity to reassess her health-promotion efforts.

SCREENING HIGH-RISK AND MODERATE-RISK WOMEN FOR BREAST CANCER

For women whose lifetime risk of being diagnosed with breast cancer is at least 20%, screening recommendations are less controversial.[14,15] These high-risk women include those with known high risk genetic mutations, those who are expected high-risk mutation carriers (family history of multiple cases of early onset breast/ovarian cancer), those with a personal history of high-dose radiation at a young age,[16,17] and those with a personal history of atypical hyperplasia, lobular carcinoma in situ (LCIS), or ductal carcinoma in situ (DCIS). The benefits of screening with any test generally outweigh the risks in these women because the positive predictive value of any abnormal finding is much higher than it would be in the general population. Mammography is recommended on an annual basis starting at 25 years of age or earlier as is annual magnetic resonance imaging (MRI) (except in women with DCIS or perhaps LCIS). The fact that MRI emits no ionizing radiation is very important for women who carry BRAC1 or BRAC2 mutations because those mutations result in deficient homologous-recombination DNA repair.[18] A Markov Monte Carlo decision analysis in BRCA1 mutation carriers confirmed that annual combined mammography and MRI screening provided the highest rate of cancer detection, the greatest life-expectancy gain, and the greatest breast cancer mortality reduction; but it also confirmed that more than 80% of screened high-risk women would have at least one false-positive finding during their lives. More than one-third of screened women would be recalled 4 or more times for further evaluation and more than a quarter would require biopsies that would reveal benign disease.[19] In settings where breast MRI is not available, the addition of ultrasound to mammography has been shown to increase cancer detection rates as well as false-positive findings.[20] Monthly BSE and semiannual CBE may not have demonstrated benefits in monitoring high-risk women but are usually recommen-ded (or at least are not opposed) by experts. One survey of women with *BRAC1* and *BRAC2* mutations reported that 94% strongly agreed or agreed that CBE is an impor-tant way to detect breast cancer, and almost all who performed BSE at least occasion-ally thought it provides an important connection to the health care team.[21]

Recommendations for screening moderate-risk women (those with a lifetime risk of breast cancer of 15%–20%) are poorly defined. Some authorities have suggested that MRI screening may be appropriate, especially if the woman understands the implica-tions of a false-positive result as well as the high rate of false positivity with MRI.[22] Others have found that screening mammography of women in their 40s is justified only when a woman's risk is double that of age-matched women in the general pop-ulation.[23] The threshold for screening with digital mammography is higher, requiring a 4.3-fold increased risk because of the higher rates of false positivity especially with women in their 40's.[23] CBE has been recommended every 6 to 12 months along with annual mammography and encouragement of BSE but without much formal anal-ysis either of the balance between benefits and risks or of cost-effectiveness.[24]

GENERAL POPULATION SCREENING

Women who are identified to have a lifetime risk for breast cancer less than 15% compose the largest group and are the focus of ongoing controversies for each of the classic screening tests: BSE, CBE, and mammography.

BSE Controversies

Before imaging techniques were available, BSE was encouraged because most palpable lesions were identified by the patients themselves.[25,26] Women who regularly practiced BSE presented with smaller tumors, which were less likely to have nodal involvement.[27–30] Even though the ability of BSE to reduce breast cancer deaths was at best inconsistently documented,[31–34] for years no harm was seen in encour-aging its use. However, a study of 132,079 women who performed well-supervised and intensively reminded monthly BSE for 5 years, 10-year outcomes were compared with those of a control group of 133,085 women with no BSE. BSE showed no reduc-tion in cancer deaths but was associated with nearly a doubling of the detection of benign lesions that required further evaluation.[35,36] The study investigators concluded: "Women who choose to practice BSE should be informed that its efficacy is unproven and that it may increase their chances of having a benign breast biopsy."[35] This study caused the American Cancer Society to change its position from a positive recom-mendation to a neutral position saying: "It is acceptable for women to choose not to do BSE or to do BSE occasionally."[37] Similar findings were reported in a WHO study in Russia.[38] As a result, the WHO recommends SBE for raising awareness among women at risk rather than as a screening method. Despite the general consistency in lack of enthusiasm for BSE, some health care providers still argue that for young women, encouragement of proper BSE is warranted and should be advocated as a quality health maintenance practice to better detect palpable masses.[39]

CBE Controversies

The limitations of CBE have been documented for years; studies have reported the sensitivity of CBE to be 40% to 69% and its specificity to be 88% to 99%.[40] These estimates were verified in a recent study of 752,081 women aged 40 years or older, which showed that the sensitivity of CBE for breast cancer detection was 58.8% and the specificity was 93.4%.[41]

However, the use of CBE continues to be supported because mammography typically misses 10% to 15% of palpable masses and because the addition of CBE to mammography increases the number of cancers detected by screening. In one study, cancer detection was increased with CBE by an additional 7.4 cancers per 1000 screenings.[24,42] The incremental value of adding CBE was also documented in a Canadian study of 290,230 women in which the sensitivity of the combination of CBE and mammography was higher than the sensitivity of mammography alone (94.6% vs 88.6%). Once again however, women who were screened with both CBE and mammography had higher rates of false-positive results (12.4%) than women who had mammography alone (7.4%).[43]

Efforts have been made to enhance clinician skills by standardizing the CBE techniques. The hope has been that this might improve the ability of CBE to reduce breast cancer deaths, especially in women younger than the age at which they would have routine mammographic screening.[44]

Mammography Screening Controversies

The most heated arguments about breast cancer screening for the general population are about the appropriate role of mammography. The questions asked about mammography may vary for different age groups, but the first fundamental question that must be answered is this: does screening mammography reduce breast cancer deaths? It may seem strange to raise the issue when the public is so convinced that mammography plays a pivotal role, but the data deserve a fresh review.

Assuming that the benefit for mammography can be demonstrated, the decisions about the proper role for mammography will depend on the answers to 2 additional qualitative questions that are rarely addressed: (1) Does mammography do more good than harm? To answer this pivotal question, it is necessary to define what is meant by each of those terms. (2) What level of financial investment in screening for breast cancer is acceptable and what analytic approach should be adopted to answer that question?

Does mammographic screening reduce breast cancer mortality?

Mammography was the first screening test that offered the possibility that breast cancer could be detected before it became a systemic disease. The smallest cell mass able to be detected by mammogram is 1 mm in diameter; that represents a mass that takes 7 years to develop from the mutation of the initial cancer cell. Between 1 mm (the threshold for mammographic detection) and 1 cm (the average size of the lesion detected by CBE), 10% to 15% of breast cancers metastasize. The existence of this "mammographic window" or "sojourn time"[24] combined with the understanding that the smaller the size of the lesion detected, the greater the woman's survival rate, together justified the initial enthusiasm for mammography. Clinical trials showed that the sensitivity of screening mammography ranged between 83% and 95%, with specificity rates between 90% and 95%. The variability in these estimates reflects the significant differences in the effectiveness of mammography seen in women of different ages. A meta-analysis showed that among women in their 50s, mammographic screening reduces breast cancer deaths by 14%; that benefit increases to 32% among women screened in their 60s.[45]

Not all of the early studies were of equal value. In a 2011 Cochrane review, the investigators rated the quality of the 8 eligible trials; only 3 were found to have adequate randomization.[46] Interestingly, the trials with adequate randomization did not find *any* effect of screening mammograms on breast cancer deaths after 10 years (relative risk [RR] 1.02, 95% confidence interval [CI] 0.95–1.10). The investigators showed, however, that mortality rates were statistically significantly lower when the results of the suboptimally randomized studies were included (RR 0.81, 95% CI 0.74–0.87). The investigators concluded that mammography probably reduced breast cancer mortality by about 15%; but that number represented a very small risk reduction for the average woman, amounting to as absolute risk reduction of only 0.05% per year.[46]

Others have argued that the Cochrane review process excluded observational studies and, therefore, missed a rich source of information about the positive impact of mammography.[47] For example, a case-control study in Western Australia reported 49% average reduction in breast cancer deaths among screened women compared with unscreened women.[48]

Is mammographic screening responsible for the recently observed reduction in breast cancer deaths?

To the question about the value of mammography, researchers have asked if the decrease seen in breast cancer deaths since the introduction of mammography should be attributed to screening or the development of better treatments. The claim for mammography's contribution to breast cancer survival is supported by many indirect studies. One such study reported that 75% of breast cancer deaths occurred among the 20% of women who were not screened.[49] However, it is possible that there may have been selection bias in that type of analysis. For example, women who do not or cannot access screening services may have similar problems with accessing or using treatment services.

A recent analysis compared breast cancer mortality rates in screened women (women older than 40 years) with those rates in women who were not screened only because they were too young (younger than 40 years). The researchers found that since the introduction of screening mammography for women aged 40 years and older, breast cancer mortality in that older-age screened group decreased by 28%, but the breast cancer mortality rates for younger women, who were not routinely screened, declined by 42%. The investigators suggested that the observed decrease in breast cancer deaths in screened age groups may be more appropriately attributed to better treatment than to early detection resulting from mammography.[50]

On the other hand, a consortium of investigators developed 7 independent statistical models of US breast cancer incidence and mortality to determine what proportion of the total reduction in breast cancer death rates should be attributed to screening, to initial treatment, or to adjuvant therapy from 1975 to 2000. The consortium found considerable variability in the estimate of the credit caused by screening, ranging from Norwegian 28% to 65% (median 46%).[51] A Norwegian study compared outcomes of women from counties where mammography was offered more recently (1996–2005) with outcomes in counties where mammography had not been available. The investigators calculated that screening itself accounted for about one-third of the observed reduction in breast cancer mortality.[52] The WHO concluded that mammography screening can reduce breast cancer mortality by

20% to 30% only under very specific conditions: in women 50 years of age or older in high-income countries in which screening coverage is more than 70%.[53]

What harm does mammography do?

Is mammography safe? The risk of exposure to radiation from mammography repeated over a woman's life is modest. Eighty-six cancers would be induced and 11 deaths would result from radiation-induced breast cancer for every 100,000 women screened 23 times (screened annually from 40 to 55 years of age and biennially from 57 to 74 years of age).[54] Models show that these risks, although not insignificant, are outweighed by the expected mortality reduction routinely attributed to mammographic screening.

But questions about safety must go beyond this. Safety must also consider the risks of each of the following:

- False-positive test results which cause unnecessary follow-up testing as well as possible misdiagnosis which could lead to unnecessary treatment (mastectomy, chemotherapy, radiation)
- False-negative results, which may *falsely* reassure patients or their clinicians
- Clinically insignificant results (overdiagnosis): finding a cancer (and treating it) that would never have caused the woman any problems
- Incurable results: finding a cancer and initiating therapy that causes significant morbidity without any benefit

What is the extent of false-positive mammographic studies? The magnitude of the problem of false-positive results is proportional to the number and frequency of scans performed. Because there are no offsetting benefits to the women from these follow-up tests and there are real medical, psychological, and financial risks associated with them, the false-positive results must be viewed as causing harm to the women being screened. If women are screened annually from 40 to 69 years of age, estimates are that, on average, each woman would be expected to have more than 2 abnormal test results during her screening and that 16% of screened women would require unnecessary biopsies.

Does mammographic screening overdiagnose breast cancer? Implementation of an effective screening tool is expected to increase the rate of detection of early disease initially; but that early surge should be followed later by a decline in late-stage disease, although the overall detection rate should not change.[55] That pattern did not happen after the introduction of mammography. Using the Surveillance, Epidemiology, and End Results database, researchers compared breast cancer rates for the period 1970 to 1978 (when mammographic screening rates were about 30%) were compared with breast cancer rates in 2006 to 2008 (when 70% of women were being screened). At baseline, the rates of early breast cancer and the rates of late-stage disease were almost equal (112 per 100,000 women and 102 per 100,000 women, respectively). By 2006 to 2008, early stage disease rates had more than doubled to 234 per 100,000, but late-stage disease decreased only slightly to 94 per 100,000. The author concluded that mammographic screening had reduced late-stage disease by only 8 per 100,000, but resulted in the diagnosis of an additional 122 early stage breast cancer. These 122 women/100,000 were then treated for early stage disease that would not have progressed to late-stage disease. The investigator estimated that with mammographic screening, more than 1 million clinically insignificant breast cancers had been diagnosed and treated during that time and that mammography had virtually no impact on the incidence of metastatic disease.[50]

The 2011 Cochrane review pointed out that the number of mastectomies and lumpectomies was greater in the screened group (RR = 1.31, CI 95% 1.22–1.42) and the use of radiation therapy similarly increased. The investigators calculated that for every 2000 women who are screened annually for 10 years, 1 woman would have her life prolonged, but 10 women would be treated unnecessarily for benign lesions thought on mammography to possibly represent cancer.[56]

In the United Kingdom, where women are screened every 3 years, it was reported that 19% of breast cancer diagnosed by mammographic screening and treated would never have caused the woman any problems; further, it has been estimated that for every 43 breast cancer deaths that would be prevented per 100,000 women who were screened, another 129 women would be harmed.[57] Based on randomized studies, another published estimate placed the magnitude of overdiagnosis of breast cancer by mammography at 25%.[56] Two recent studies have suggested that mammographic breast cancer screening could be causing more harm than good after 10 years.[46,58] The American Cancer Society has now formally taken the position that screening for breast cancer can come with a real risk of overtreating many small cancers while missing cancers that are deadly.

What are our goals in mammographic screening?

Arguments about when to start mammographic screening in the general population and how frequently to screen women often result from disagreements about the fundamental purpose of mammography. **Table 3** displays the explicit tradeoffs that were considered by the USPSTF when it made its 2009 recommendations.[40] The USPSTF numbers highlight the impact of the fundamental question of whether our goal in mammographic screening should be to maximize the number of breast cancer deaths prevented or to maximize the number of years of life gained by early detection and treatment. If the latter is the goal, clearly it would be important to include younger women in the screened pool because they would be expected to live longer.[59] Every analysis shows that delaying routine mammography until 50 years of age is the most effective approach for reducing breast cancer deaths, but initiating screening at 40 years of age is more effective in increasing the number of life-years gained with screening.[59] Until we as a society determine what goal we wish to achieve, disputes will continue.

Table 3
Trade-off in screening seen in USPSTF analysis

Ages (y)	Mammograms per 1000 Women	Mortality Reduction (%)	Cancer Deaths Averted per 1000 Women	Life-years Gained per 1000 Women	False-Positive Results per 1000 Women	Unnecessary Biopsies per 1000 Women
Biennial screening						
40–69	13,865	16	6.1	120	1250	88
50–69	8944	15	5.4	99	780	55
Annual screening						
40–69	27,583	22	8.3	164	2250	158
50–69	17,759	20	7.3	132	1350	95

Data from Mandelblatt JS, Cronin KA, Bailey S, et al. Effects of mammography screening under different screening schedules: model estimates of potential benefits and harms. Ann Intern Med 2009;151(10):744.

The USPSTF's recommendation to exclude 40 year olds in the general population from routine screening rested on several points: the lower risk faced by women in their 40s for developing breast cancer, lower mammographic sensitivity in that age group, and higher false-positive rates. This analysis also introduced considerations of efficacy into the calculation. For example, 1904 women need to be screened in their 40s to prevent one breast cancer death, whereas that number is only 1339 for women in their 50s and 377 for women in their 60s.[24]

What analysis should be used to decide the details of screening age and frequency?
Regardless of the primary objective chosen for mammographic screening, the reality is that there are only limited resources available to invest in any given health problem. We need to carefully assess the contributions made by each screening strategy using appropriate comparisons. The most expensive strategies are always the most effective, but they are rarely the most efficient.[60] Therefore, it is not appropriate to compare *total* numbers in **Table 3** for each option. For example, the 164 years of life that would be gained per 1000 women screened annually for 30 years (from 40–69 years of age) cannot just be compared with the 99 years of life gained per 1000 women imaged every other year from 50 to 69 years of age without considering the cost and harms associated with each of those screening protocols. The most appropriate analysis is to compare *incremental* benefits and risks. Assume we start with the USPSTF's recommendations as a base case in which 8944 scans done per 1000 women save 5.4 lives per 1000 women and gain 99 years of life per 1000 scans. The questions would then be how much *more* benefit would be added by including young women in the biennial screening option by performing an additional 4921 scans. The answer is that 0.7 more lives per 1000 more scans per 1000 women would be saved and 21 years of life per 1000 scans per 1000 women would be gained. This answer demonstrates obvious diminishing returns for investment in more scans. The yield is even lower when the USPSTF's recommendations are compared with the American College of Obstetricians and Gynecologists' annual screening starting at 40 years of age. The recommendations for additional 18,639 scans required per 1000 women would only reduce mortality by 2.9 lives and increase years of life by 65 years (or 1.27 days per scan). As the USPSTF pointed out, their approach saved 81% as many lives as the annual and early screening recommendations with less than one-third the numbers of scans.

What can we do with the available information?
The USPSTF's recommendations for general population screening meet the standards of do no harm and cost-effective use of resources, but many clinicians fear adopting them because of patient resistance to such change. Advocacy groups, the media, and even postal stamps encourage the use of mammography.[61] Small increases in breast cancer cases make headlines; when it was found that metastatic breast cancer cases in women aged 25 to 39 years increased from 1.53 per 100,000 women in 1976 to 2.9 per 100,000 in 2009, headlines proclaimed that breast cases rates had doubled without noting how rare the event still was. The impact that advocacy groups have on women's perception of breast cancer itself and the ability of screening tests to modify that risk is truly impressive. Celebrity endorsements of testing and personal testimonials ("mammography saved my life") are usually very powerful even if they are not true; such claims are growing in numbers as the pool of breast cancer survivors is continuously growing.

Against this backdrop of potentially overstated benefits, we must also present patients with an estimate of their risks. The risks (harms) associated with virtually every screening test are generally proportional to the number of tests performed, whereas the incremental benefits of tests drop precipitously as the numbers of tests increase.

This balance must be communicated to women as they consider their own screening options. One analysis points out that women view breast screening as a way of avoiding potential regret; they highly value the reassurance normal results provide. They seemed to be aware of false positives and the anxiety they cause but not of overdiagnosis.[62]

The information can be somewhat complicated and the tradeoffs overwhelming. As an example, the following has been offered as model counseling to provide women in this situation:

> "Mammography is an X-ray of the breasts that may help to detect breast cancer before symptoms develop. It has been shown to reduce the risk of dying from breast cancer by 15%. It does not detect all breast cancers but typically detects between 60% and 90% of breast cancers. Your chance of getting breast cancer in your 40's is approximately 1 in 70 women, Approximately 1 in 10 women have screening mammograms will need further evaluation, such as additional mammogram images. In most cases, this additional testing will be negative for cancer. Would you like to proceed with mammographic screening?"[24]

Although this is complete information, it may be difficult for women to absorb and digest on the spot.

For women who respond to mathematical arguments, the numbers speak clearly. A woman's lifetime risk of dying from breast cancer is approximately 3%. Screening her every other year from 50 to 74 years of age with 12 scans lowers that risk to 2.3%. Screening her every year from 40 to 84 years of age with 44 scans lowers her risk another 0.5% to 1.8%.[63] By more than tripling the numbers of scans required, the risks of false-positive results increase dramatically, with little additional benefit.

Insight about how to approach this problem may come from another study from New Zealand. Primary care providers asked their patients aged 50 to 70 years 2 questions: (1) How many breast cancer deaths do you think would be prevented if a group of 5000 women were to be screened for 10 years? (2) What is the minimal acceptable benefit (chance that the testing would save your life) that you would accept before you agreed to undergo breast cancer screening?[64] Not surprisingly, more than 90% of women overestimated the numbers of deaths (2–15) prevented by screening. Even more interesting, however, was the fact that if women knew how small the real effectiveness of breast cancer screening in preventing breast cancer deaths is, 70% said they would not submit to it.

Using focus groups, researchers recently explored women's awareness of possible overdiagnosis with mammography and the impact that knowledge would have on their intentions to seek screening. Most women had no prior knowledge of this problem; but with counseling, the investigators reported that women came to understand it. At the rates currently estimated for overdiagnosis (up to 30%), women said they would remain committed to routine screening. At higher rates, women said they might continue to be screened, but they would consider the possibility of overdiagnosis when they were deciding about treatment.[65]

IMPLICATIONS FOR THE FUTURE

Breast cancer is projected to continue to increase as the US population ages; the total number of cases of breast cancer is expected to increase by 30% by 2030, with some of the largest increases expected among ethnic groups that have not traditionally accessed routine health care and breast cancer screening.[6] With health care dollars limited and the need for services expanding, we will need to invest our resources prudently. This will require significant changes and new approaches, but education can be pivotal.[66] A key element will be to work with each individual woman to estimate on an ongoing basis what her personal short-term and lifetime risks for breast cancer are. Women with only background risks can be reassured by that knowledge, and it is hoped that they will understand why screening guidelines are designed to protect their health by simultaneously maximizing the effectiveness of screening and minimizing the real harms associated with testing.

As new understanding of the pathophysiology of various subtypes of breast cancer improves, new risk factors may emerge to change risk classification and influence screening recommendations.[67] In the future, new technology may also change the balance between risk and benefits. Screening recommendations must be dynamically reassessed over time.

REFERENCES

1. American College of Obstetricians-Gynecologists. Practice bulletin no. 122: breast cancer screening. Obstet Gynecol 2011;118(2 Pt 1):372–82.
2. Warner E. Clinical practice. Breast-cancer screening. N Engl J Med 2011; 365(11):1025–32.
3. Anderson BO, Yip CH, Smith RA, et al. Guideline implementation for breast healthcare in low-income and middle-income countries: overview of the Breast Health Global Initiative Global Summit 2007. Cancer 2008;113(Suppl 8): 2221–43.
4. WHO breast cancer prevention and control. Available at: http://www.who.int/cancer/detection/breastcancer/en/. Accessed March 1, 2013.
5. Wilson JM, Jungner J. Principles and practice of screening for disease. Geneva: World Health Organization; 1968.
6. Centers for Disease Control and Prevention (CDC). Vital signs: racial disparities in breast cancer severity–United States, 2005-2009. MMWR Morb Mortal Wkly Rep 2012;61(C45):922.
7. Macciò A, Madeddu C. Obesity, inflammation, and postmenopausal breast cancer: therapeutic implications. ScientificWorldJournal 2011;11:2020–36.
8. Barlow WE, White E, Ballard-Barbash R, et al. Prospective breast cancer risk prediction model for women undergoing screening mammography. J Natl Cancer Inst 2006;98(17):1204–14.
9. Smith-Warner SA, Spiegelman D, Yaun SS, et al. Alcohol and breast cancer in women: a pooled analysis of cohort studies. JAMA 1998;279(7):535–40.
10. Zhang S, Hunter DJ, Hankinson SE, et al. A prospective study of folate intake and the risk of breast cancer. JAMA 1999;281(17):1632–7.
11. Guerra CE, Sherman M, Armstrong K. Diffusion of breast cancer risk assessment in primary care. J Am Board Fam Med 2009;22(3):272–9.
12. Sabatino SA, McCarthy EP, Phillips RS, et al. Breast cancer risk assessment and management in primary care: provider attitudes, practices, and barriers. Cancer Detect Prev 2007;31(5):375–83.
13. Sontag A, Wickerham L, Ni X, et al. Estimated risk of invasive breast cancer in postmenopausal women with and without family history of the disease. Menopause 2011;18(5):515–20.
14. Petrucelli N, Daly MB, Feldman GL. Hereditary breast and ovarian cancer due to mutations in BRCA1 and BRCA2. Genet Med 2010;12(5):245–59.
15. National Cancer Institute. PDQ: genetics of breast and ovarian cancer. Available at: http://cancer.gov/cancertopics/pdq/genetics/breast-and-ovarian/health professional/. Accessed March 1, 2013.

16. Taylor AJ, Taylor RE. Surveillance for breast cancer after childhood cancer. JAMA 2009;301(4):435–6.
17. Oeffinger KC, Ford JS, Moskowitz CS, et al. Breast cancer surveillance practices among women previously treated with chest radiation for a childhood cancer. JAMA 2009;301(4):404–14.
18. Foulkes WD. Traffic control for BRCA1. N Engl J Med 2010;362(8):755–6.
19. Lee JM, Kopans DB, McMahon PM, et al. Breast cancer screening in BRCA1 mutation carriers: effectiveness of MR imaging–Markov Monte Carlo decision analysis. Radiology 2008;246(3):763–71.
20. Berg WA, Zhang Z, Lehrer D, et al, ACRIN 6666 Investigators. Detection of breast cancer with addition of annual screening ultrasound or a single screening MRI to mammography in women with elevated breast cancer risk. JAMA 2012; 307(13):1394–404.
21. Spiegel TN, Hill KA, Warner E. The attitudes of women with BRCA1 and BRCA2 mutations toward clinical breast examinations and breast self-examinations. J Womens Health (Larchmt) 2009;18(7):1019–24.
22. Mainiero MB, Lourenco A, Mahoney MC, et al. ACR appropriateness criteria breast cancer screening. J Am Coll Radiol 2013;10(1):11–4.
23. van Ravesteyn NT, Miglioretti DL, Stout NK, et al. Tipping the balance of benefits and harms to favor screening mammography starting at age 40 years: a comparative modeling study of risk. Ann Intern Med 2012;156(9):609–17.
24. Griffin JL, Pearlman MD. Breast cancer screening in women at average risk and high risk. Obstet Gynecol 2010;116(6):1410–21.
25. Gould-Martin K, Paganini-Hill A, Casagrande C, et al. Behavioral and biological determinants of surgical stage of breast cancer. Prev Med 1982;11(4): 429–40.
26. Tamburini M, Massara G, Bertario L, et al. Usefulness of breast self-examination for an early detection of breast cancer results of a study on 500 breast cancer patients and 652 controls. Tumori 1981;67(3):219–24.
27. Senie RT, Rosen PP, Lesser ML, et al. Breast self-examination and medical examination related to breast cancer stage. Am J Public Health 1981;71(6):583–90.
28. Feldman JG, Carter AC, Nicastri AD, et al. Breast self-examination, relationship to stage of breast cancer at diagnosis. Cancer 1981;47(11):2740–5.
29. Mant D, Vessey MP, Neil A, et al. Breast self examination and breast cancer stage at diagnosis. Br J Cancer 1987;55(2):207–11.
30. Foster RS Jr, Lang SP, Costanza MC, et al. Breast self-examination practices and breast-cancer stage. N Engl J Med 1978;299(6):265–70.
31. Foster RS Jr, Costanza MC. Breast self-examination practices and breast cancer survival. Cancer 1984;53(4):999–1005.
32. Ogawa H, Tominaga S, Yoshida M, et al. Breast self-examination practice and clinical stage of breast cancer. Jpn J Cancer Res 1987;78(5):447–52.
33. Huguley CM Jr, Brown RL, Greenberg RS, et al. Breast self-examination and survival from breast cancer. Cancer 1988;62(7):1389–96.
34. Locker AP, Caseldine J, Mitchell AK, et al. Results from a seven-year programme of breast self-examination in 89,010 women. Br J Cancer 1989;60(3): 401–5.
35. Thomas DB, Gao DL, Self SG, et al. Randomized trial of breast self-examination in Shanghai: methodology and preliminary results. J Natl Cancer Inst 1997; 89(5):355–65.
36. Thomas DB, Gao DL, Ray RM, et al. Randomized trial of breast self-examination in Shanghai: final results. J Natl Cancer Inst 2002;94(19):1445–57.

37. Smith RA, Saslow D, Sawyer KA, et al, American Cancer Society High-Risk Work Group; American Cancer Society Screening Older Women Work Group, American Cancer Society Mammography Work Group, American Cancer Society Physical Examination Work Group, American Cancer Society New Technologies Work Group; American Cancer Society Breast Cancer Advisory Group. American Cancer Society guidelines for breast cancer screening: update 2003. CA Cancer J Clin 2003;53(3):141–69.

38. Semiglazov VF, Manikhas AG, Moiseenko VM, et al. Results of a prospective randomized investigation [Russia (St. Petersburg)/WHO] to evaluate the significance of self-examination for the early detection of breast cancer. Vopr Onkol 2003;49(4):434–41 [in Russian].

39. Fancher TT, Palesty JA, Paszkowiak JJ, et al. Can breast self-examination continue to be touted justifiably as an optional practice? Int J Surg Oncol 2011;2011:965464.

40. US Preventive Services Task Force. Screening for breast cancer: U.S. Preventive Services Task Force recommendation statement. Ann Intern Med 2009; 151(10):716–26. http://dx.doi.org/10.1059/0003-4819-151-10-200911170-00008 W-236. [Erratum appears in Ann Intern Med 2010;152(10):688; Erratum appears in Ann Intern Med 2010;152(3):199–200].

41. Bobo JK, Lee NC, Thames SF. Findings from 752,081 clinical breast examinations reported to a national screening program from 1995 through 1998. J Natl Cancer Inst 2000;92(12):971–6.

42. Barton MB, Harris R, Fletcher SW. The rational clinical examination. Does this patient have breast cancer? The screening clinical breast examination: should it be done? How? JAMA 1999;282(13):1270–80.

43. Chiarelli AM, Majpruz V, Brown P, et al. The contribution of clinical breast examination to the accuracy of breast screening. J Natl Cancer Inst 2009;101(18): 1236–43.

44. Saslow D, Hannan J, Osuch J, et al. Clinical breast examination: practical recommendations for optimizing performance and reporting. CA Cancer J Clin 2004;54(6):327–44.

45. Nelson HD, Tyne K, Naik A, et al, U.S. Preventive Services Task Force. Screening for breast cancer: an update for the U.S. Preventive Services Task Force. Ann Intern Med 2009;151(10):727–37, W237–42.

46. Gøtzsche PC, Nielsen M. Screening for breast cancer with mammography. Cochrane Database Syst Rev 2011;(1):CD001877.

47. Berg WA. Benefits of screening mammography. JAMA 2010;303(2):168–9.

48. Nickson C, Mason KE, English DR, et al. Mammographic screening and breast cancer mortality: a case-control study and meta-analysis. Cancer Epidemiol Biomarkers Prev 2012;21(9):1479–88.

49. Cady B, Michaelson JS, Chung MA. The "tipping point" for breast cancer mortality decline has resulted from size reductions due to mammographic screening. Ann Surg Oncol 2011;18(4):903–6.

50. Bleyer A, Welch HG. Effect of three decades of screening mammography on breast-cancer incidence. N Engl J Med 2012;367(21):1998–2005.

51. Berry DA, Cronin KA, Plevritis SK, et al, Cancer Intervention and Surveillance Modeling Network (CISNET) Collaborators. Effect of screening and adjuvant therapy on mortality from breast cancer. N Engl J Med 2005;353(17):1784–92.

52. Kalager M, Adami HO, Bretthauer M, et al. Overdiagnosis of invasive breast cancer due to mammography screening: results from the Norwegian screening program. Ann Intern Med 2012;156(7):491–9.

53. IARC world cancer report 2008. Lyon International Agency for Research on Cancer. Available at: http://www.iarc.fr/en/publications/pdfs-online/wcr/. Accessed March 5, 2013.
54. Yaffe MJ, Mainprize JG. Risk of radiation-induced breast cancer from mammographic screening. Radiology 2011;258(1):98–105.
55. Esserman L, Shieh Y, Thompson I. Rethinking screening for breast cancer and prostate cancer. JAMA 2009;302(15):1685–92.
56. Welch HG, Black WC. Overdiagnosis in cancer. J Natl Cancer Inst 2010;102(9): 605–13.
57. Nelson R. Breast screening saves lives, but at a cost, UK panel concludes. Available at: http://www.medscape.com/viewarticle/773552. Accessed March 3, 2013.
58. Raftery J, Chorozoglou M. Possible net harms of breast cancer screening: updated modelling of Forrest report. BMJ 2011;343:d7627.
59. Mandelblatt JS, Cronin KA, Bailey S, et al, Breast Cancer Working Group of the Cancer Intervention and Surveillance Modeling Network. Effects of mammography screening under different screening schedules: model estimates of potential benefits and harms. Ann Intern Med 2009;151(10):738–47.
60. Ahern CH, Shen Y. Cost-effectiveness analysis of mammography and clinical breast examination strategies: a comparison with current guidelines. Cancer Epidemiol Biomarkers Prev 2009;18(3):718–25.
61. Woloshin S, Schwartz LM. The benefits and harms of mammography screening: understanding the trade-offs. JAMA 2010;303(2):164–5.
62. Hersch J, Jansen J, Irwig L, et al. How do we achieve informed choice for women considering breast screening? Prev Med 2011;53(3):144–6.
63. Mandelblatt JS, Cronin KA, Berry DA, et al. Modeling the impact of population screening on breast cancer mortality in the United States. Breast 2011; 20(Suppl 3):S75–81.
64. Hudson B, Zarifeh A, Young L, et al. Patients' expectations of screening and preventive treatments. Ann Fam Med 2012;10(6):495–502.
65. Hersch J, Jansen J, Barratt A, et al. Women's views on overdiagnosis in breast cancer screening: a qualitative study. BMJ 2013;346:f158.
66. Murphy AM. Mammography screening for breast cancer: a view from 2 worlds. JAMA 2010;303(2):166–7.
67. Cancer Genome Atlas Network. Comprehensive molecular portraits of human breast tumours. Nature 2012;490(7418):61–70.

Current Breast Imaging Modalities, Advances, and Impact on Breast Care

Evelyn M. Garcia, MD[a,c,*], Erik S. Storm, DO[b,c],
Lisa Atkinson, RTR(M), BS[b], Eileen Kenny, MD[b,c],
Lisa S. Mitchell, MBA[a]

KEYWORDS

- Breast MRI • Mammography • Tomosynthesis • Elastography • BSGI • PEM

KEY POINTS

- Mammography remains the screening modality of choice for breast cancer, with wide availability and standardized quality measures. Measurable advantages in detection for digital mammography have been found in women with dense parenchyma only.
- Advanced imaging modalities are available for problem solving and guidance of breast interventions. These modalities include ultrasonography and magnetic resonance imaging.
- Advances in imaging capabilities in the form of new reconstruction algorithms and techniques of image acquisition for existing technologies have the potential to improve sensitivity, specificity, and accuracy of staging. These techniques include tomosynthesis, elastography, diffusion imaging, and perfusion imaging.
- Molecular imaging in the form of positron emission tomography (PET) and PET/computed tomography has been used in the staging and restaging of breast cancer. The innovations of breast-specific gamma imaging and positron emission mammography have potential for detection of cancer before the neovascularization stage, detection of ductal carcinoma in situ (DCIS) before development of calcifications, and identification of breast cancer in dense breast parenchyma.

INTRODUCTION

Mammography is a commonplace screening procedure undergone by millions of women in America on an annual or biennial basis or at other intervals, depending on patient preference or physician recommendation. According the US Centers for

---

Disclosures: The authors have nothing to disclose.
[a] Department of Radiology, Carilion Roanoke Memorial Hospital, Carilion Clinic, 1906 Belleview Avenue, Roanoke, VA 24014, USA; [b] Breast Care Center, Carilion Roanoke Community Hospital, Carilion Clinic, 101 Elm Avenue, Roanoke, VA 24013, USA; [c] Virginia Tech Carilion School of Medicine, 2 Riverside Circle, Roanoke, VA 24016, USA
* Corresponding author. Department of Radiology, Carilion Roanoke Memorial Hospital, Carilion Clinic, 1906 Belleview Avenue, Roanoke, VA 24014.
E-mail address: emgarcia@carilionclinic.org

Obstet Gynecol Clin N Am 40 (2013) 429–457
http://dx.doi.org/10.1016/j.ogc.2013.05.002
0889-8545/13/$ – see front matter © 2013 Elsevier Inc. All rights reserved.

Disease Control and Prevention (CDC), more than 20 million mammograms occur annually from physician office visits, whereas another 2.3 million take place in outpatient hospital settings.[1] Further, more than 67% of women aged 40 years and older have had a mammogram in the last 2 years.[2] However, mammography is seldom thought of by patients or the public except during times of increased visibility, such as Breast Cancer Awareness Month, or, on a more personal level, when a reminder letter arrives in the mail.[3] Patients and/or the public consider even less the adjunctive and problem-solving imaging procedures available throughout the nation. Many of the adjunctive and problem-solving procedures are widely available in rural as well as metropolitan areas; whereas others are still evolving in showing mortality or clinical benefit and are unavailable because of geographic, economic, or other access barriers. Overshadowing the success of mammography in reducing morbidity and mortality are the limitations inherent to this readily accessible screening procedure.[4,5]

MAMMOGRAPHY

Mammography has been the gold standard for early detection of breast cancer for the last 50 years. The first mammography unit used for population-based screening was developed in 1960 by Dr Philip Strax. Research into the usefulness of using radiation to image the breast began as early as 1913, with the imaging of surgical breast specimens.[6] Continued research, equipment improvements, and clinical-based trials such as the Swedish Twin Counties Trial have set the stage for modern mammography.[7] Despite controversy during the last 20 years, mammography remains the best screening tool for the early detection of breast cancer.

Analog, film-screen mammography was the most consistent means of image acquisition. However, in 2003, the US Food and Drug Administration (FDA) approved the use of the first digital mammography units.[8] These units provided clear advantages in film archiving, efficiency, and interpretation of dense breasts. At first, the cost was prohibitive for many facilities. During this evolutionary phase of mammography, patients may have received either analog or digital imaging.

Analog and digital mammography use low-dose x-rays to acquire images of the breast, compression to improve visualization, and produce two-dimensional (2D) images of the breast. Four basic views are obtained: craniocaudal (CC) and mediolateral oblique (MLO) of each breast, but this is where the similarities end.

Analog mammography uses x-ray film as the imaging receptor as well as the storage medium.[8] A photosensitive chemical layer bonded to the media is exposed by the x-rays passing through the breast tissue. Unlike digital mammography, analog mammography images must undergo a chemical process to develop the latent image and to fix it to the film. Analog images, also referred to as hardcopy films, are viewed by projecting light through the film. The film cannot be manipulated for better visualization, making areas of increased density more difficult to interpret. Analog mammography also limits patient throughput. Processing and quality checking of images by the technologist add, on average, 15 minutes per patient examination.

Digital mammograms are acquired by using detector technology. Photosensitive detectors integrated into the mammography unit are exposed and the resultant electronic signal is translated into the digital image. Storing of images is managed via a picture archiving and communication system (PACS). These images are referred to as soft copy images and can be retrieved from PACS electronically for future comparison. As digital images are reviewed on workstations, images may be manipulated to improve conspicuity of densities, masses, and calcifications. Patients notice 1 specific difference with the acquisition of digital images. As the image is acquired, it transmits to a computer monitor in the mammography room. The image is available for quality review by the technologist within seconds, reducing examination time significantly.

Quality control is required on both analog and digital units and is regulated through the American College of Radiology (ACR), or state accrediting body, and the FDA. For analog mammography, standards were set by the ACR. This standardization occurred with the passing of the Mammography Quality Standards Act (MQSA) in 1992. The FDA allowed the individual equipment vendors to set their own criteria, limits, and frequency for quality testing of the equipment. Although these tests are similar across different vendors, each has unique, vendor-specific requirements.

Digital mammography has been reported to have increased sensitivity compared with analog/film-screen mammography in dense breasts of 70% compared with 55%, respectively (**Fig. 1**).[9] Dense breasts, those containing greater than 50% fibroglandular tissue, make cancer detection difficult because of the similarity in density of indicators of breast cancer such as calcifications, asymmetric densities, and masses to benign fibroglandular tissue on mammography (**Figs. 2 and 3, Table 1**).

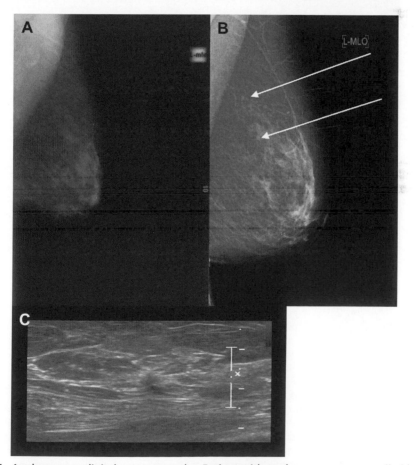

Fig. 1. Analog versus digital mammography. Patient with analog mammogram called back for asymmetric density seen on CC view only, which proved to be normal tissue. A significant finding on digital mammogram (*B*) of two 5-mm invasive ductal carcinomas (*arrows*) not seen on analog (*A*) imaging. Corresponding ultrasound is seen of one of these cancers (*C*).

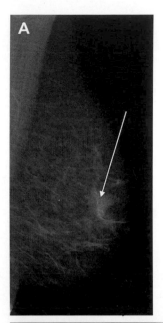

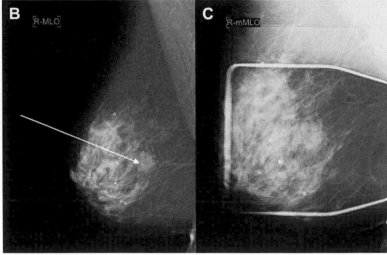

Fig. 2. Digital images: fatty versus dense. (*A*) Biopsy-proven invasive ductal carcinoma (*arrow*) in a fatty breast. (*B, C*) Biopsy-proven invasive ductal carcinoma (*arrow*) in a dense breast.

Sensitivity and specificity are two of the measures used to determine the accuracy with which breast imaging radiologists interpret mammography. Sensitivity is defined as the number of BI-RAD (Breast Imaging-Reporting and Data System) category 4 and 5 interpretations with a positive biopsy result (true-positive). Specificity is defined as the number of BI-RADS 1 to 3 interpretations that are true-negative.[10] Studies have shown that, for analog and digital mammography, the sensitivity and specificity are similar except for a small subset of patients. These are (1) women who have dense breast tissue, (2) women who are less than age 50 years, and (3) women who are premenopausal or perimenopausal.[11,12] **Table 3** shows sensitivity and specificity

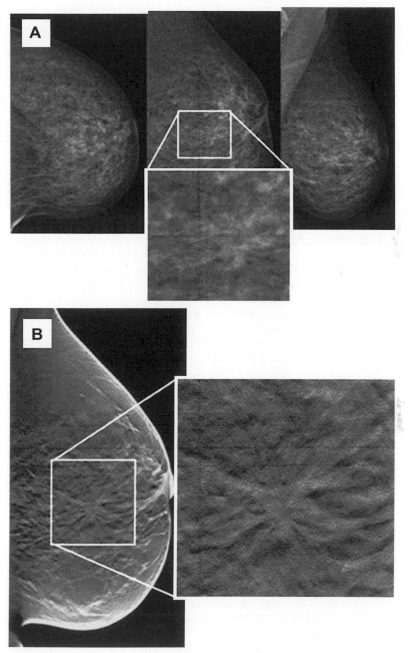

Fig. 3. Full-field digital mammography (FFDM), dense breast parenchyma, architectural distortion (*A*); digital breast tomosynthesis of same lesion (*B*). (*From* Diekmann F, Bick U. Breast tomosynthesis. Semin Ultrasound CT MR 2011;32(4):285; with permission.)

Table 1 BI-RADS density categories		
BI-RADS Category	Description	Percentage Dense Parenchyma
1	Fatty	0–24
2	Scattered fibroglandular density	25–49
3	Heterogeneously dense	50–74
4	Extremely dense	75–100

Data from Yaffe MJ. Measurement of mammographic density. Breast Cancer Res 2008;10:209.

ranges for analog and digital mammography as well as the newest technology, tomosynthesis.[11,13] As of December 3, 2012, MQSA National Statistics show that 89% of all mammography facilities have added full-field digital mammography (FFDM) to their breast imaging arsenal.[14]

The American Cancer Society (ACS), the ACR, the Society of Breast Imaging (SBI), and the American College of Obstetrics and Gynecology (ACOG) guidelines recommend yearly screening mammography in all women 40 years of age and older (**Table 2**). The ACS reports a 30% reduction in mortality from breast cancer directly linked to screening mammography.

Ordering the correct imaging study is important so that cancers are not missed. Family history and symptoms must be considered when ordering a screening mammogram. A woman must be asymptomatic to obtain a screening mammogram and an order is not required. If a patient is symptomatic, she needs a diagnostic mammogram. When a diagnostic work-up is ordered, the standard 2 mammographic views will be obtained, plus additional views such as spot compression or magnification as needed, and possibly ultrasound may also be performed. Specific information regarding the location of concern is necessary to ensure evaluation of the correct area and avoid a false-negative report.

TOMOSYNTHESIS

Digital breast tomosynthesis (DBT) is a low-dose x-ray data set of the compressed breast obtained over a limited arc and mathematically reconstructed into a series of sections for display. Image acquisition is similar to current FFDM in that the breast is stabilized through paired compression plates and an x-ray source is used to expose a digital detector. The data set acquired may be displayed at varying slice thicknesses or in slabs. There is currently 1 tomosynthesis unit approved for clinical use by the FDA, the Hologic Selenia Dimensions (Hologic, Bedford, Mass; 2/11/11, http://www.fda.gov/Radiation-EmittingProducts/MammographyQualityStandardsActand Program/FacilityCertificationandInspection/ucm114148.htm). The unit is capable of acquiring DBT and FFDM views, which is the current procedure approved by the FDA.[15]

Digital breast tomosynthesis is of greatest potential value in women with dense breast tissue that has been shown to be an independent risk factor for breast carcinoma and is associated with decreased sensitivity and specificity in mammography, film screen, and digital (see **Table 3**).[16,17] DBT overcomes the main limitation of mammographic imaging: the reduction of a three-dimensional (3D) structure to a 2D image.[18–20] Radiation dose is similar to FFDM. Digital breast tomosynthesis average radiation dose per exposure is 0.7 and 0.82 mGy (range 0.28–1.42 mGy) compared with FFDM at 0.6 and 1.2 mGy (range 0.2–2.4 mGy) for CC and MLO views,

Table 2
Screening recommendations

Risk	Factor	Age to Begin Screening[a] (y)	Frequency	Mammography	Ultrasound	MRI
Average	None	40	Annual	+	−	−
Increased	First-degree relative with proven BRCA1 or BRCA2	30	Annual	+	−	+
	≥20% lifetime risk for breast cancer	30, or 10 y before age of diagnosis in youngest affected relative	Annual	+		
	Premenopausal breast cancer in mother or sister	30, or 10 y before age of diagnosis in youngest affected relative	Annual	+		
	Personal history of mantle radiation received between ages of 10 and 30	8 y after receiving treatment	Annual	+		
	Biopsy-proven lobular neoplasia, atypical ductal hyperplasia, ductal carcinoma in situ, invasive breast cancer, or ovarian cancer	From time of diagnosis	Annual	+		

[a] Screening should not begin before the age of 25 years.

Data from Lee CH, Dershaw DD, Kopans D, et al. Breast cancer screening with imaging: recommendations from the Society of Breast Imaging and the ACR on the use of mammography, breast MRI, breast ultrasound, and other technologies for the detection of clinically occult breast cancer. J Am Coll Radiol 2010;7(1):18–27.

respectively.[9,18,21] Mean glandular dose of DBT of 4.1 ± 0.3 mGy compared favorably with combined FFDM and digital spot compression views (DSCV) of 4.69 ± 1.7 mGy.[22]

The DBT technique improves identification of lesions in dense breast parenchyma by diminishing the obscuration caused by superimposition of normal tissues of similar density.[22–25] This improvement is achieved through the focus of each reconstructed image being limited to a specific volume of breast tissue with smearing of out-of-plane tissue. Benefits of DBT include better depiction of tumor margins with more accurate characterization of margin type and mass size,[23,24] and it has been shown to have a better correlation of tumor size with breast ultrasonography compared with FFDM.[25,26] In addition, Wallis and colleagues[21] found that it increases sensitivity,

Table 3 Digital versus film mammography		
	Sensitivity (%)	Specificity (%)
Film-screen mammography	66	92
Full-field digital	70	92
Tomosynthesis	93	84–86

Data from Arnold L. Sensitivity and specificity of digital vs. film mammography. Internet Journal of Academic Physician Assistants 2010. Available at: http://archive.ispub.com/journal/the-internet-journal-of-academic-physician-assistants/volume-7-number-2/sensitivity-and-specificity-of-digital-vs-film-mammography.html#sthash.lbqEvEth.dpbs. Accessed January 24, 2013.

specificity, and reader confidence, which fulfills 2 important goals of a screening technology: increased conspicuity of malignancies and ability to detect malignancies currently missed by FFDM.[25]

DBT has also been shown in studies by Skaane and colleagues[25] and Bernardi and colleagues[27] to have superior detection rate and confidence for architectural distortion related to breast cancer (see Figs. 2 and 3). Clinical performance studies have shown decreased recall rates and/or increased sensitivity to asymmetric densities, architectural distortions, and nodules with regular margins for DBT compared with FFDM. It did not affect performance for intrinsically suspicious lesions such as stellate opacities and calcifications.[9,23]

DBT has not been shown to be superior to FFDM in detection or characterization of calcifications and, in several studies, has been inferior with sensitivities of 75% and 84%, respectively.[15,28–32] This limitation is thought to be related to several characteristics of DBT image sets. There is the perceptual challenge of thin slices obscuring the distribution of calcifications. Clusters of calcifications may be reduced to a few calcifications visible in any given image slice.[25,33] The smearing effect of tomography may diminish the ability to characterize the shape of calcifications through decreased spatial resolution.[30,31] The increased time of acquisition required for DBT, 5 to 10 seconds, increases the risk of motion artifact obscuring subtle microcalcifications.[30,31] These limitations may be balanced through review of image slabs, which have the potential to better depict configuration and distribution of calcification clusters in 3D space.[18,30]

Other limitations of DBT are review time and the attendant reader fatigue. The image data sets are larger than current FFDM, with increase in interpretation time of up to 100%, range 70% to 100%.[21,30,34,35] These limitations may be balanced by the potential increase in reader confidence and decrease in recall rates, which have yet to be studied.

Comparability with mammographic spot views for decision making in the diagnostic setting has been shown. In 1 study, all readers showed slightly better mass visibility though only 1 reached statistical significance.[36] In this study, an additional 1.8 cancers were detected at the cost of 1.3 additional false-positive biopsies. A second study also showed increased lesion conspicuity on DBT compared with DSCV.[22] This finding again suggests the potential to decrease patient recall rates and benign biopsies with the attendant patient anxiety and its associated negative effects.[9,21–23,36]

The primary benefit of DBT to patients lies in the combination of improved detection and confidence. Additional benefits are the potential to decrease recall rates, as noted earlier, with the decreasing mean glandular dose through obviating additional views,[19,23,25,33] decreasing the benign biopsy rate through decreased false-positives,[23] and more accurate BI-RADS classification at initial screening or diagnostic examination.[25]

ULTRASOUND

Research using ultrasound to detect breast masses began in the 1950s with John Wild.[37] His intention was to create a medical device that could be used to screen for breast masses. He did not know that, in 2012, the FDA would approve the first automated breast ultrasound device for use in screening of patients with mammographically dense breasts.[38] The use of ultrasound as an adjunctive diagnostic tool to mammography is well documented. However, the use of ultrasonography as a screening tool remains an active topic of research.[39]

Ultrasound uses high-frequency sound waves to produce images of the breast. This technology is currently used to differentiate the cystic versus solid nature of a clinically palpable mass or to further characterize abnormal mammographic findings. Ultrasound characteristics are used to differentiate benign masses from malignant and for axillary evaluation for pathologic lymphadenopathy.

To date, there are no known age-related algorithms that are considered standard of care for women presenting with a palpable lump. Most palpable lumps in young women are benign. They are usually fibroadenomas or normal, hormonally stimulated fibroglandular tissue.[40] Confirmation with further imaging studies is recommended to fully assess the nature of the clinical finding. Breast imagers use clinical history, mammography, ultrasound, and physical examination findings to arrive at a diagnosis.

In our practice, if a woman less than 30 years of age presents with a palpable lump, her first imaging study is ultrasound. Mammography is rarely used because of the radiation risk, albeit minimal, in young breast tissue. If a suspicious finding is seen on ultrasound or a palpable abnormality is clinically suspicious but ultrasonographically occult, mammography is performed to search for suspicious findings. In patients 30 years of age and older presenting with a palpable mass, diagnostic mammography is performed with potential ultrasound to complete imaging characterization.

Ultrasound characteristics suspicious for malignancy include spiculated margins, dimensions that are taller than wide, posterior acoustic shadowing, and/or associated calcifications. Benign characteristics include hyperechogenicity, oval or elliptical shape, dimensions that are wider than tall, well-circumscribed margins, and a thin echogenic capsule (**Fig. 4**). The presence of internal echoes indicates that a mass is solid, but it still could be benign in nature. Recommendations for the next steps are included in the imaging report. They may range from return to screening (BI-RADS 1 or 2), short-term follow-up (BI-RAD 3), cyst aspiration, or biopsy (BI-RAD 4/5).

Directed, or diagnostic, breast ultrasound, as described earlier, is currently the most common practice. However, with the introduction of breast density legislation in many states, the role of ultrasound in breast cancer screening may soon change. Legislation passed or pending in 19 states requiring women to receive a letter of notification if they have dense breast tissue is a source of confusion for patients and physicians. An additional complication is that most insurance companies do not recognize screening breast ultrasound. Helping patients weigh the risks associated with screening ultrasound, potentially higher callback and false-positive rates, with the benefit of increased cancer detection is critical.[41]

Screening ultrasound has yet to be recommended by the ACR, but studies show that the addition of ultrasound to screening mammography in women with dense breasts can increase the sensitivity up to 96.6%.[42] Although screening mammography is known to detect 4 to 5 cancers/1000 women screened per year, this number has been shown to almost double with an additional 3.25 cancers/1000 women when screening ultrasound is added in women with dense breast parenchyma and no other risk factors.[43,44] Berg and colleagues[44] found similar numbers (additional 4.2

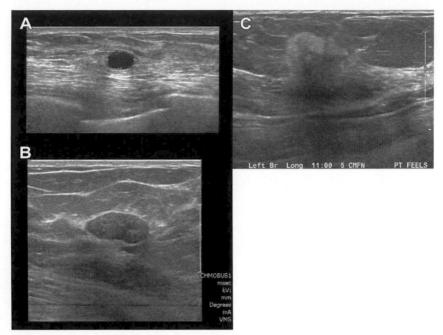

Fig. 4. Ultrasound imaging: Simple cyst (*A*). Biopsy-proven fibroadenoma (*B*). Biopsy-proven invasive ductal carcinoma (*C*).

cancers/1000 women) when ultrasound is added to screening mammography in high-risk patients. These cancers were found to be small and node-negative. At our center, we find that approximately 40% of women have dense breasts, which is consistent with the reported national average of 41%.[45]

Ultrasound is also used for guidance of interventional procedures such as cyst aspiration, abscess drainage, and biopsy (**Figs. 5** and **6**). These procedures can be performed by the breast intervention practitioner or radiologist. At our breast center, the breast surgeons have entrusted us to perform 99% of the interventional procedures recommended so that a precise, definitive surgery can be performed for

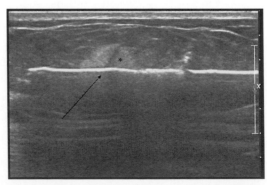

Fig. 5. A biopsy needle (*arrow*) traversing a breast mass (*asterisk*) surrounded by normal breast parenchyma.

A

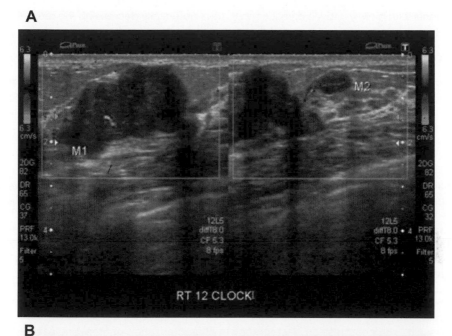

B

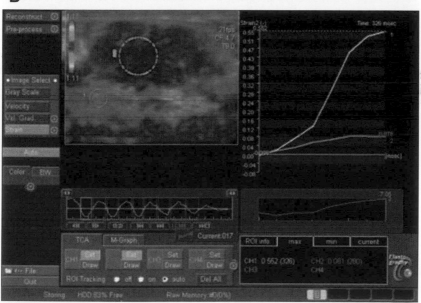

Fig. 6. Gray-scale ultrasound image of invasive ductal carcinoma and satellite lesion (*A*), and elastogram and strain map of the same two lesions (*B*). (*From* Mansour SM, Omar OS. Elastography ultrasound and questionable breast lesions: does it count? Eur J Radiol 2012;81(11):3239; with permission.)

patients with biopsy-proven breast cancer, thus potentially decreasing the reexcision rate.

ULTRASOUND ELASTOGRAPHY

Breast cancer is generally harder than normal tissue. This quality forms the basis for physical examination.[46] Elastography takes advantage of the differences in the physical properties of elasticity and strain of masses and normal tissue to create diagnostic information.[47] Elasticity is the tendency of a tissue to resume its original size and shape.[48] Strain is the level of change in size or shape in response to external compression.[48,49] Strain within tissue is smaller in harder tissues such as breast cancer.

There are 2 different types of elastography. Shear-wave elastography (SWE) is accomplished when "an acoustic pressure wave induces slow-moving lateral waves within the tissue, and the speed of propagation of the shear wave is proportional of the square root of the tissue's elastic modulus."[50] Strain or compression elastography ultrasonography (CEU) is performed using pressure applied by the ultrasound operator or from a patient source such as respiration or cardiac pulsation. Images are based on measuring the relative tissue displacement induced.[51] This qualitative measure is limited by user-related differences in transducer placement, pressure applied, and reproducibility. SWE overcomes these limitations because the pressure is produced and the velocity changes are measured by the same ultrasound transducer.[51,52]

Results with compression elastography in characterization of breast masses were promising with similar sensitivity and specificity compared with conventional ultrasonography (**Table 4**).[49,53] Images were produced as color maps of the compression results superimposed on the gray-scale images. Malignant masses were stiffer than benign masses and appeared larger than the corresponding mass seen on conventional morphologic ultrasound images.[54,55] This finding is also seen in SWE (see **Figs. 5** and **6**)[56] and may be caused by a local effect of the mass on the surrounding tissues, desmoplastic reaction in the surrounding tissues, or tumor extent beyond what is visible on ultrasonography.[54,55]

SWE is performed using a conventional linear array probe, allowing it to be integrated into the ultrasound examination with real-time acquisition of the data.[57] This method also increases reproducibility of the results.[52] On average, 3 to 5 minutes are added to the time of the examination. Unlike compression elastography, reliability does not depend on the operator.[50,53,57–59] In addition, the data acquired are quantitative, based on the velocity of the induced wave in tissue.[47,51]

Initial studies indicated potential benefits of decreasing unnecessary biopsies and short-interval follow-up.[49,60] This potential gain is greatest for the BI-RADS category

Table 4 Results of compression elastography					
Modality	Sensitivity (%)	Specificity (%)	Accuracy (%)	PPV (%)	NPV (%)
CEU	70.1	95.7	88.2	87.1	88.5
CEU	86.5	89.8	88.8[a]	—	—
SWE	97	83	91	88	95
Ultrasonography	87	78	83	84	82
SWE	97	83	—	88	95

[a] Cutoff point between BI-RADS3 and 4; positive cutoff value 50 kPa.
Data from Refs.[50,54,59,61]

3 and 4 lesions. The information provided by morphologic studies and elastography are complementary and can improve management of BI-RADS category 3 and 4a lesions, in particular.[46,50,56] Elastography results should not be used to downgrade BI-RADS 4b, 4c, or 5 lesions or change management in BI-RADS category 2 lesions (**Table 5**).[56,57,59,61] As with other imaging modalities, the most suspicious finding should drive management. The combination of morphologic ultrasonography and SWE increases specificity and enables earlier diagnosis of breast cancer.[54] Information acquired with elastography having significant potential as a determinant in future management decisions includes mean stiffness, maximum stiffness, and shape of the zone of stiffness.[56]

Elastography of calcified lesions may provide some diagnostic value. Elastogram stiffness of tissue with mammographic calcifications differed for benign and malignant lesions. Benign lesions had lower stiffness than malignant. Ductal carcinoma in situ (DCIS) has intermediate stiffness between invasive carcinoma and benign lesions. Benign proliferative lesions, nonproliferative lesions, and DCIS were all less stiff than invasive carcinomas.[62]

Elastography may also prove useful in patients undergoing neoadjuvant chemotherapy. SWE has shown a higher response rate to neoadjuvant chemotherapy in patients with soft malignancies than those with hard malignancies.[63] Tumor stiffness is a characteristic of the extracellular matrix. Increased extracellular matrix is involved in tumor progression.[63] Because SWE is a quantitative measure of tissue stiffness that is directly related to extracellular matrix, measurable changes in stiffness may serve as indicators of tissue response.

There is a limitation caused by overlap in elasticity between benign and malignant lesions.[64] False-negative findings occur in DCIS, early stages of invasive carcinoma, carcinomas with large necrotic areas, mucinous carcinomas, papillary carcinomas, and medullary carcinomas.[49,52,57,60,64] False-positive findings occur in stiff benign processes such as fibroadenoma, surgical scar, postradiation skin thickening, inflammation, fat necrosis, hyalinized fibroadenomas, and fibrocystic lesions; and processes of questionable malignant potential such as papilloma and radial scars.[52,57,58]

Factors found to limit sensitivity and specificity of elastography included depth of the lesion from the skin, breast thickness at the location of the lesion, and lesion diameter greater than transducer length. Thick breast tissue attenuates both sound and elastic waves. As noted earlier, compression elastography also has limited reproducibility caused by operator-induced differences and the lack of quantitative

Table 5 BI-RADS categories		
BI-RADS Category	**Descriptive Comment**	**Likelihood of Malignancy (%)**
1	Negative	—
2	Benign finding	—
3	Probably benign	<2
4a	Low suspicion of malignancy	>2 to <10
4b	Intermediate suspicion of malignancy	>10 to <50
4c	Moderate suspicion of malignancy	>50 to <95
5	Highly suggestive of malignancy	>95

Data from Mansour SM, Omar OS. Elastography ultrasound and questionable breast lesions: does it count? Eur J Radiol 2012;81(11):3234–44.

information, which lead to significant variability in image acquisition and interpretation.[46–48,53,56,58,59]

BREAST MAGNETIC RESONANCE IMAGING

Contrast-enhanced breast magnetic resonance imaging (BMRI) is a valuable adjunctive tool for both breast cancer screening and for further evaluation of known breast disease, without the risks of additional ionizing radiation. Clinical practice guidelines published by the ACR outline current indications for the use of BMRI (Refer to **Table 2**).[13]

The value of BMRI as an adjunctive screening modality in the high-risk patient population has been firmly established over the past few decades. Breast cancers in the high-risk group often occur at a younger age and are frequently of a higher grade and clinical stage at diagnosis than those detected by screening mammography alone. The sensitivity of BMRI in high-risk women approaches 100% for invasive breast disease versus less than 50% for mammography. This population can include young patients and those with dense breast tissue.[65,66] A recently published, large, multicenter, randomized study by Berg and colleagues[67] compared the benefit of adjunctive breast ultrasound and BMRI in 2809 high-risk women with dense breasts. The sensitivity of combined mammography, ultrasound, and BMRI was 100%, with a specificity of 65%. For mammography only, sensitivity and specificity were 52% and 91% respectively.

BMRI following biopsy-proven diagnosis of breast cancer is a common part of the multimodality approach to breast cancer treatment and helps to determine extent of disease and guide local therapy (**Fig. 7**). BMRI has been shown to be an accurate method for staging the size and anatomic extent of breast cancer, including identification of unsuspected additional areas of malignancy.[68] It has been reported that 63% of breast cancers originally thought to be of limited extent by conventional imaging and clinical breast examination have been shown to be multifocal on subsequent detailed pathologic analysis of mastectomy specimens.[69] Recent investigations have shown that a patient with a newly diagnosed breast cancer has a 6% risk of occult synchronous ipsilateral breast cancer and a 4% risk of occult contralateral breast cancer.[70] Knowledge of the potential extent of tumor is desirable to guide surgical management, which aids in reaching the goal of reduced reexcision for positive margins and potentially reduces cancer recurrence from unexcised tumor burden.

In cases of breast conservation therapy with positive surgical margins, postoperative BMRI has been shown to be accurate for assessment of residual tumor burden, indicating incomplete excision.[71] This knowledge can then guide reexcision, especially in cases in which there are no malignant calcifications seen on postoperative mammography.

Patients with locally advanced breast cancer are frequently treated with preoperative (neoadjuvant) chemotherapy, which has been shown to reduce tumor burden and enable the surgeon to subsequently obtain clear margins. BMRI has been shown to have a sensitivity of 63% and specificity of 91% for determination of pathologic complete response, with a strong correlation between residual tumor sizes measured by magnetic resonance imaging (MRI) compared with size reported on surgical pathology.[72]

Technological advances have enabled rapid, simultaneous imaging acquisition of both breasts while maintaining high spatial and temporal resolution. The procedure is that a woman's breasts are immobilized in a high-resolution imaging coil. Multiple sequences are obtained to accentuate the intrinsic T1 and T2 tissue properties. T1

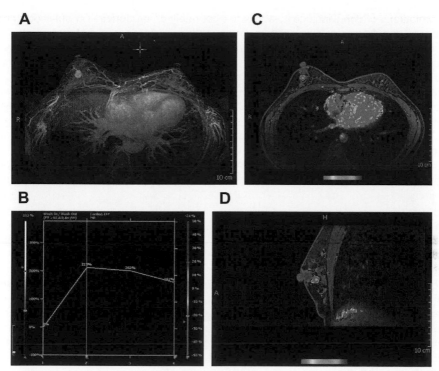

Fig. 7. Screening MRI examination on a 45-year-old woman at increased risk of breast cancer. Her mammogram 6 months ago was dense, but otherwise negative. (*A*) Axial maximum intensity projection image showing a 1.2-cm round mass in the retroareolar right breast. This mass remained occult on the follow-up diagnostic mammogram (*B*). Kinetic analysis of the red area of the mass showing rapid initial enhancement, followed by progressive washout on the subsequent time points. This washout pattern, and the rim-enhancement pattern are both highly suspicious for malignancy. Subsequent biopsy showed intermediate-grade invasive ductal carcinoma. (*C*) Axial and (*D*) sagittal T1 first postcontrast subtracted images.

imaging is performed before administration of gadolinium contrast and followed by at least 3 dynamic sequential postcontrast series. Characteristic enhancement is associated with breast malignancy because of several factors, including tumor angiogenesis and increased vascular permeability.

The interpretation of BMRI is best done by comparison with other multimodality imaging, most notably the most recent screening mammogram. Areas of asymmetric enhancement are analyzed on both a morphologic (structural) and kinetic (functional) basis, using well-established criteria. The examination is typically given an overall BI-RADS final assessment category as in mammograms, as described elsewhere in this article. A BI-RADS 4 or 5 finding indicates that a suspicious abnormality has been detected. In this case a second-look ultrasound may be performed to determine whether an abnormality can be confirmed. The reported success of MRI-directed (second-look) ultrasound is variable, but a recent meta-analysis of 16 studies shows that 64% of suspicious lesions on MRI were subsequently identifiable by ultrasound.[73] If the suspect lesion cannot confidently be identified, MRI guidance can be used for biopsy or localization for surgical excision.

Limitations of BMRI include its ability to accurately characterize very small (<5 mm) lesions, and frequent false-positive findings that may lead to further diagnostic work-up. The sensitivity and specificity of the examination are compromised when there is a significant degree of hormonally mediated background parenchymal enhancement, which can decrease the conspicuity of small areas of malignancy. The optimum timing for performance of the BMRI examination for a premenopausal routine screening patient is in the proliferative phase of her menstrual cycle. The premenstrual week should be avoided.

Contraindications to the procedure include those referred to later, the presence of a pacemaker and/or other non–MR-compatible implanted device, and documented adverse reaction to gadolinium-containing contrast. Relative contraindications include morbid obesity and the inability to lie prone and remain still for the duration of the examination.

PERFUSION MRI

There are 2 techniques for perfusion MRI: arterial spin labeling (ASL) and T2*-weighted sequences. Both rely on the perfusion parameters of the microvascular environment. Parameters affecting perfusion include vascular permeability (K_{trans}), the rate of contrast escape from the extracellular extravascular space into the plasma compartment (K_{ep}), and the extracellular vascular compartment (ve). These characteristics differ between normal breast tissue and breast lesions because of tumor-related angiogenesis. The microvascular changes caused by tumor angiogenesis are more directly reflected in dynamic than in static imaging.[74]

T2*-weighted imaging is a first pass contrast-enhanced technique requiring high temporal resolution. Signal intensity decreases in the first 30 seconds after contrast administration.[75] The tumor microvascular environment causes loss of signal because of the effect of the high volume of contrast on the surrounding tissue magnetic environment, which is the result of disruption of spin phase coherence caused by the local gradient that is created.[76]

ASL is a noncontrast technique to assess tissue perfusion.[77] This technique may prove valuable in patients with contraindications to gadolinium-based contrast material such as in renal insufficiency, liver disease, and cardiac dysfunction. ASL uses magnetic-labeled arterial blood water as an endogenous tracer to measure perfusion. The higher perfusion characteristics of most breast cancers are measurably different from the lower rate of surrounding normal breast tissue. These differences are reflected in the higher vascular permeability and capillary density that are seen on histologic evaluation of fast-growing breast tumors.[78]

Perfusion imaging may also prove a useful adjunct to morphologic MRI in assessment of early treatment response. Accurate evaluation before surgery offers the potential to avoid unnecessary procedures in patients with favorable prognoses.[79] Correlation between anatomic MRI and histopathology in determination of residual tumor is unreliable and may lead to missed detection in up to 30% of patients.[79] The functional analysis provided by perfusion imaging could differentiate chemotherapy responders from nonresponders more reliably. Treatment-related changes in tumor vessels with the attendant changes in blood volume, vessel density, and permeability are measurable after 1 to 2 cycles of neoadjuvant chemotherapy. K_{trans} and K_{ep} correlate with prognostic factors of high histologic grade, high nuclear grade, and estrogen receptor (ER) negativity. ve correlates with the prognostic factors of high histologic grade and ER negativity. These parameters correspond with anatomic dynamic contrast-enhanced MRI correlation of early enhancement and washout curve with high histologic grade and ER negativity.[78]

Any condition that influences blood perfusion may affect K_{trans}, including cardiac output and hypertension. These do not affect K_{ep}, which reflects return of leaked contrast back into the intravascular space, indicating capillary permeability. For this reason, K_{ep} may provide a more accurate indication of tumor capillary permeability. Decreased ve in tumors may be explained by the smaller extracellular space and disorganized microarchitecture related to the high cellular density of malignant tumors.

There are multiple potential limitations to perfusion MRI. There is overlap in perfusion imaging characteristics between benign and malignant lesions, which may lead to misclassification of DCIS and hypervascular benign masses. Also, coverage and signal/noise ratio are sacrificed for high temporal resolution. Because breast tumors are frequently difficult to differentiate from surrounding tissue in the absence of contrast material, localization before performing perfusion imaging may be compromised. Hormone therapy (HT) causes significant increases in breast tissue perfusion, which may affect detection and characterization of lesions on perfusion MRI,[80] which is of concern because of the increased risk of breast cancer in women on HT.[81-84] The cause for these changes may be related to the histaminelike effect of estrogen, increasing microvascular permeability and inducing vasodilation and the mitogenic effect of progesterone, which might increase metabolic activity. BMRI readers differ on whether or not to stop HT before imaging. This decision is site specific based on the location of image acquisition.

DIFFUSION MRI

Diffusion-weighted MRI (DWI) is a noncontrast technique measuring the random brownian motion of water molecules in vivo. DWI reflects the microscopic cellular environment in tissues. It is affected by multiple local tissue factors including cell density, cell organization, membrane permeability, blood flow, extracellular space, intercellular macromolecules, directionality of cellular structures, and microvessel density.[85-89] Diffusion-weighted images are paired with apparent diffusion coefficient (ADC) maps.

ADC measures alteration of mean diffusivity of water molecules by reflecting the level of restriction to diffusion. Therefore, ADC correlates inversely with barriers to diffusion.[86,90] It is affected by diffusion and perfusion, reflecting molecular diffusivity and blood microcirculation, including capillary density, intravascular flow, and cardiac pulsation.[85,87,91] Because of this, diffusion imaging is performed with a minimum of 2 acquisitions using different b values. Selection of b value is important in limiting the microcirculation effect, which may increase ADC in malignant tumors. Low b values are less diffusion weighted because they use less gradient and may yield higher ADC because of a greater reflection of the local perfusion environment on the measured value. High b values are mainly affected by diffusion.[92] No consensus exists as to how many or which b values should be used in BMRI or what constitutes the appropriate diagnostic thresholds.[93,94] Increasing the number of b values used increases the specificity of DWI, but this comes at the cost of increased imaging time.

Malignant tumors have increased cellular density with decreased interstitial space, which increase barriers to diffusion.[94] For these reasons, diffusion is inversely correlated with cellularity and cell membrane integrity.[95] Diffusion-weighted images show high signal intensity in structures with dense cellularity because of retention of signal. Vascular structures, low-cellular-density foci, and normal breast tissue produce fewer barriers and a more organized microstructural environment allowing greater signal loss as excited protons move more quickly in the volume imaged. The inverse proportionality of ADC yields a low-intensity or dark focus in densely cellular structures such as carcinomas.

Because of its sensitivity to the microstructural environmental factors listed earlier, DWI has the potential to increase the specificity of BMRI. It also has the potential to expand its use to patients with contraindications to gadolinium-based MRI contrast material (discussed earlier) and those with known allergies to contrast.

DWI also has potential for evaluation of response to neoadjuvant chemotherapy. Mammography, ultrasonography, dynamic contrast-enhanced MRI, and clinical palpation may not accurately provide early assessment of tumor response because of the late manifestations of morphologic changes.[90] Morphologic evaluations frequently overestimate residual tumor and have limited correlation with histopathologic response. Early assessment of response to treatment is important in treatment planning and management of patients with breast cancer. DWI changes may be observed after 1 cycle in responders and could help differentiate responders from nonresponders to neoadjuvant chemotherapy (NAC). Increases in ADC after NAC are related to cell damage, compromised cell membranes, and increased fractional volume of the interstitial space caused by apoptosis and cell loss.[90] These changes begin to occur within 24 hours of treatment.

There are limitations of DWI and ADC measurements. False-positives may be seen in highly cellular benign lesions and in association with processes causing local changes in magnetic susceptibility.[96,97] Examples are highly cellular intraductal papillomas and fibroadenomas. False-negatives may be seen in lesions with low cellularity such as mucinous carcinoma, carcinomas with necrotic foci, and in areas of hemorrhage. DWI is also limited by low spatial resolution.[95] The higher the b value, the higher the diffusion weighting and the lower the resolution.

MOLECULAR IMAGING

The multiple modalities used primarily for the morphologic depiction of the breast are discussed earlier with emerging applications based on the physiology of cancer and currently used successfully in other imaging subspecialties. Molecular imaging differs in that it is based on the physiology of the cell targeted for imaging. Carrier molecules are chosen specifically for their ability to become incorporated into functional cells through existing physiologic pathways. Breast-specific gamma imaging (BSGI) and positron emission mammography (PEM) are two of these molecular imaging procedures that have shown promise. The ultimate role of molecular imaging in breast disease is uncertain because of the systemic nature of the radiolabeled carrier molecules and delivery of the associated radiation dose to nontarget tissues.

BSGI

99m Technetium (99mTc) is a gamma-emitting radioisotope used commonly in nuclear medicine/molecular imaging. When coupled to methoxyisobutylisonitrile (sestamibi), it is used for cardiac imaging and is FDA approved for breast scintigraphy.[98] Identification of the potential for breast cancer imaging was accidental, because of unexpected visualization of foci of breast activity on images of patients undergoing cardiac nuclear studies. 99mTc Sestamibi is a lipophilic agent that is taken up by cytoplasmic mitochondria. Mitochondrial density is an indicator of cellular proliferation that is taken advantage of in BSGI.[99]

BSGI is performed with high-resolution gamma detectors configured to optimize resolution in the breast. Images obtained are similar to and directly comparable with the standard CC and MLO views of x-ray mammography. Early studies noted limitations in resolution related to use of standard gamma cameras that suffered from suboptimal configuration for close approximation to the breast and lower resolution scintillation crystal technology.[100]

After injection, 99mTc sestamibi concentrates in proliferating cells, creating a focus of increased activity that is translated by the gamma detectors into a hot spot on the images produced. The typical BSGI study comprises 4 to 10 images composed of slices of a set thickness through the breast. Acquisition is sequential and has a duration of 5 to 10 minutes for each breast. There is still some question as to the optimal time after injection for imaging. Early imaging may reflect the hypervascular nature of malignancies, whereas delayed imaging benefits from the clearance of radiotracer from the nontarget tissues, decreasing background and scatter radiation noise in the images.

One of the benefits of BSGI is the lack of interference of breast parenchymal density with isotope detection and image acquisition. Unlike mammography, the high-energy, 140 keV, gamma photons emitted by 99mTc are not attenuated by dense parenchyma (**Fig. 8**).[100] In an early study comparing patients with fatty and dense breasts, Khalkhali and colleagues[101] found no statistical difference in the performance of BSGI between

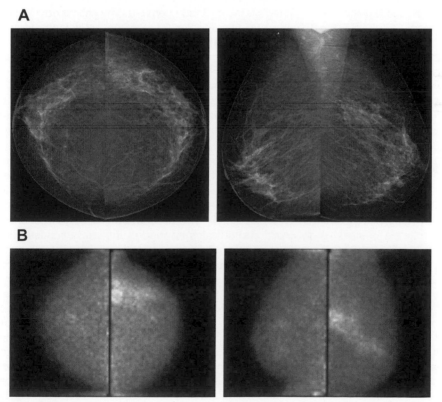

Fig. 8. FFDM BI-RADS density category 3 breasts (*A*) image matched BSGI of the same patient showing left breast DCIS (*B*). (*Courtesy of* Margaret Bertrand, MD, Greensboro, NC.)

the two groups, with sensitivities and specificities of 72% versus 70% and 80% versus 78% respectively. These ranges have improved with improvement of gamma camera geometry and tailoring the detectors for breast imaging. Current ranges for sensitivity and specificity are 89% to 98% and 77% to 93.8%, respectively.[98,102–105] In a large trial by Rhodes and colleagues[106] of women with dense breasts and increased risk for development of breast cancer, BSGI increased the detection of cancer in their cohort by 7.5 per 1000 women compared with mammography alone.

Also, there is potential for earlier diagnosis of DCIS. The typical calcifications associated with DCIS are a late finding. The physiologic nature of BSGI does not rely on the development of these calcifications.[98] Another conundrum for breast imagers is differentiation of postsurgical changes from local recurrence. The architectural distortions and scar tissue associated with breast-conserving therapy may mask the earliest morphologic indications of recurrence on mammography. The physiologic changes are evident on BSGI.[107,108] In addition, BSGI may be useful for local staging of patients with biopsy-proven breast cancer and dense breast tissue by showing multifocal or multicentric disease that is mammographically occult in patients who have contraindications for MRI.[103,104,109]

Limitations of BSGI are related to nonmalignant proliferative processes in the breast, with the most common false-positive results caused by fibroadenomas, intraductal papillomas, proliferative breast processes, and fibrocystic changes.[104,107] As noted earlier, another limitation of BSGI is the radiation dose. The National Council on Radiation Protection and Measurements (NRCP) report #60 estimates an average background radiation in the United States of 3 mSv per year. The estimated effective dose for 1 BSGI is 5.9 to 9.4 mSv, equivalent to 2 to 3 times annual background radiation for living in the United States in 1 year.[110] This is similar to the effective dose of PEM, discussed later, of 6.2 to 7.1 mSv and compares with calculated doses to breast tissue of 3.7 to 4.7 mGy for screening mammography. The difference in units is caused by the whole-body effects of systemic radiation in BSGI and PEM compared with the targeted breast exposure in mammography. For these reasons, BSGI is likely to remain an adjunctive imaging procedure until low-dose algorithms are developed and optimized.

PEM

18F-Fluorodeoxyglucose (FDG) is a positron-emitting glucose analogue capable of entering cells. During glycolysis, FDG is treated the same as glucose in the initial step of phosphorylation to FDG-6-phosphate. This product does not undergo further steps in the process of glycolysis and remains trapped in the cell. Because most malignant tumors have a higher metabolic rate than normal tissues and there is overexpression of the Glut-1 transporter in breast cancer cells, the difference in detectable positron emission allows identification of highly metabolic tissues.[111–114] This property is the basis for positron emission imaging.[112,114] PEM is based on this principle. It uses physiologic information to detect cancers that might be obscured by dense breast tissue or occult for other structural reasons.

PEM differs from whole-body positron emission tomography (PET) in that 2 planar detectors are positioned in a similar configuration as mammography detectors. Image data are collected in coincidence, which means that the 2 photons produced in a positron annihilation event must be detected by both detectors for the information to be integrated into the images produced.[113–116] Images may be acquired in the same projections as mammographic images. PEM improves spatial resolution up to 1.5 to 2.8 mm full width at half maximum compared with 5 to 7 mm full width at half maximum for whole-body PET images with reconstructed resolution of 10 to 15 mm.[116–120] Also, patient dose may be decreased 5-fold to 10-fold and acquisition decreased by 8 to 12 times.[114,121] A tumor/background uptake ratio of 6:1 is required to detect hypermetabolic tumors and for differentiation from background activity. PEM findings that indicate malignancy include focal hot spots and asymmetric breast activity.[114]

The physiologic nature of PEM imaging may allow earlier detection of small breast cancers, before neovascularization, reflected in morphologic studies as contrast enhancement characteristics, which occurs when the tumor reaches approximately 3 mm.[112,122] Hypermetabolic activity begins in tumor cells before tumor angiogenesis.[120,123] This technique may have a role in DCIS, unsuspected contralateral disease, and multifocal disease.[121,124] DCIS may not be detectable at morphologic imaging, particularly if there are no associated calcifications or neovascularity. It is frequently the cause for positive or close margins at excision. This capability has the potential to decrease reexcision rates through improved pretreatment staging.[124,125]

Additional potential indications include initial staging in newly diagnosed patients, distinguishing recurrent disease from posttreatment changes, and evaluating response to neoadjuvant chemotherapy.[115,118,119,121] One study has shown a significant correlation of prognostic indicators of cancer survival, ER, PR, and Her2 status and tumor grade with maximum PEM uptake values and lesion/background ratios, which were higher in association with ER-negative, PR-negative, and HER2-negative tumors as well as tumors with histologic Bloom-Richardson grade 3 tumors. This result only reached statistical significance in triple-negative tumors.[118]

Data suggest that PEM may detect malignant lesions 80% to 89% of the time. Specificity has been measured at 86% to 100%.[114,118,121,124,125] This finding compares favorably with mammography at approximately 81% and is similar to MRI at 86.3%. Sensitivity of PEM ranges from 90% to 95%.[115,118,120,121,125] Coordinated review of all imaging data improves diagnosis in patient with breast cancer.[125,126] False-positive results may be seen in benign hypermetabolic processes and inflammatory processes such as fibrocystic changes, fat necrosis, some fibroadenomas, ruptured cysts, and postbiopsy changes.[111,115,120,126]

Limitations to PEM are related to the geometry of the detectors and the nature of molecular imaging. Tissue close to the chest wall may be excluded. Scatter radiation from tissue outside the field of view may interfere with image reconstruction.[116,125] Poor patient positioning may also cause false-negative results.[120] The detector sensitivity decreases as distance from the center of the detectors increases,[114,117] and this causes increased noise at the edges of the images. FDG uptake is increased in dense breast tissue and may interfere with lesion detection, which may be the greatest limiting factor in the detection of small lesions with PEM.[111,113,121,126] Sensitivity of PEM is also decreased in women with large breasts, possibly because of volume averaging effect or scatter.[117,125,127] Abnormal glucose metabolism in diabetic patients may also interfere with cancer conspicuity and, therefore, detection by PEM.[121] Malignancies with low metabolic rates may produce false-negative results.[124,125] Radiation dose (estimated at 6.2 mSv whole-body radiation dose from 10 mCi of FDG comparable with a computed tomography [CT] chest-abdomen-pelvis), availability, and cost are also confounding issues in PEM.[116,126] These issues may be addressed by using PEM as a supplemental imaging examination in patients with known breast cancer following staging whole-body PET/CT, thereby obviating a second radiotracer dose.[121] Testing standards have not yet been established for PEM systems.[116]

SUMMARY

Mammography will continue as the breast cancer screening imaging study of choice for the foreseeable future. It remains the best and most accessible option throughout both metropolitan and rural communities. Ultrasound and MRI are widely available adjunctive studies for women with suspicious mammographic or clinical findings, and MRI is a screening tool for women with specific increased risks for breast cancer. There are several types of breast cancer, from ductal carcinoma to lobular carcinoma and more rarely diagnosed inflammatory breast cancer, making it a complex disease, affected by a woman's individual genetic and lifestyle risk factors. Adding to this complexity is dense breast parenchyma and overlap in clinical and imaging findings of benign and malignant lesions, which continue to confound imagers. As a result, options for diagnosis will continue to evolve and progress. This article discusses a wide variety of imaging options currently used and in development, their strengths, limitations, and potential future roles in the continuing pursuit of early breast cancer diagnosis, treatment, and follow-up.

ACKNOWLEDGMENTS

The authors thank Marjorie Gowdy for her helpful comments and editing on this article. The authors also thank Emily Gannon for assistance in formatting and preparation, and Catherine Hagan for assistance in literature searches.

REFERENCES

1. Centers for Disease Control and Prevention (CDC). National Ambulatory Medical Care Survey: 2009 summary tables. The Ambulatory and Hospital Care Statistics Branch. Available at: http://www.cdc.gov/nchs/data/ahcd/namcs_summary/2009_namcs_web_tables.pdf. Accessed February 4, 2013.
2. Centers for Disease Control and Prevention (CDC). Use of mammography among women 40 years of age and over, by selected characteristics: United States selected years 1987-2010. Available at: http://www.cdc.gov/nchs/data/hus/hus11.pdf#090. Accessed February 4, 2013.
3. Chaudhry R, et al. Effect of e-mail versus postal reminders for mammogram screening. AMIA Annu Symp Proc 2006;2006:879.
4. Nelson HD, et al. Screening for breast cancer: an update for the U.S Preventive Services Task Force. Clinical guidelines. Ann Intern Med 2009;192:10.
5. Mandelblatt JS, et al. Effect of screening mammography under different screening schedules: model estimates of potential benefits and harms. Clinical guidelines. Ann Intern Med 2009;151:738–47.
6. Gold RH, Bassett LW, Widoff BE. Radiologic history exhibit. Highlights from the history of mammography. Radiographics 1990;10:1111–31.
7. Tabar L, Bedrich V, Chen T, et al. Swedish two-county trial: impact of mammography screening on breast cancer mortality during 3 decades. Radiology 2011;260(3):658–63.
8. Digital vs. analog mammography technology spotlight. Medcompare. Available at: http://www.medcompare.com/spotlight.asp?spotlightid=32. Accessed January 4, 2013.
9. Pisano ED, Gastonis C, Hendrick E, et al. Diagnostic performance of digital versus film mammography for breast-cancer screening. N Engl J Med 2005;353(17):1773–83.

10. Evaluating screening performance in practice: assessing the performance of screening mammography. The Breast Cancer Surveillance Consortium; April 2004. Available at: http://www.breastscreening.cancer.gov. Accessed January 23, 2013.

11. Understanding breast cancer; Table 31: Digital mammography versus film mammography for breast cancer screening. Susan G. Komen for the Cure. Available at: http://www.Komen.org. Accessed January 4, 2013.

12. American College of Radiology. Practice guideline for the performance of contrast-enhanced magnetic resonance imaging (MRI) of the breast, 2008 revision. Available at: http://www.acr.org. Accessed January 4, 2013.

13. Digital breast tomosynthesis: a clinical assessment based on literature. Siemens White Paper. Available at: http://www.Siemens.com/healthcare. Accessed January 4, 2013.

14. Radiation-emitting products: MQSA national statistics. U.S. Food and Drug Administration. Available at: http://www.fda.gov/Radiation-EmittingProducts/MammographyQualityStandardsActandProgram/FacilityScorecard/ucm113858.htm. Accessed January 4, 2013.

15. Gur D, Zuley ML, Anello MI, et al. Dose reduction in digital breast tomosynthesis (DBT) screening using synthetically reconstructed projection images: an Observer Performance Study. Acad Radiol 2012;19:166–71.

16. Tagliafico A, Tagliafico G, Astengo D, et al. Mammographic density estimation: one-to-one comparison of digital mammography and digital breast tomosynthesis using fully automated software. Eur Radiol 2012;22(6):1265–70.

17. Harver JA, Bovbjerg VE. Quantitative assessment of mammographic breast density: relationship with breast cancer risk. Radiology 2004;230(1):29–41.

18. Feng SS, Sechopoulos I. Clinical digital breast tomosynthesis system: dosimetric characterization. Radiology 2012;263(1):35–42.

19. Diekmann F, Bick U. Breast tomosynthesis. Semin Ultrasound CT MR 2011; 32(4):281–7.

20. Smith A. Full-field breast tomosynthesis. Radiol Manage 2005;227:25–31.

21. Wallis MG, Moa E, Zanca F, et al. Two-view and single-view tomosynthesis versus full-field digital mammography: high-resolution X-ray imaging observer study. Radiology 2012;262(3):788–96.

22. Tagliafico A, Astengo D, Cavagnetto F, et al. One-to-one comparison between digital spot compression view and digital breast tomosynthesis. Eur Radiol 2012;22(3):539–44.

23. Zuley ML, Bandos AI, Ganott MA, et al. Digital breast tomosynthesis versus supplemental diagnostic mammographic views for evaluation of noncalcified breast lesions. Radiology 2013;266(1):89–95.

24. Engelken FJ, Sack I, Klatt D, et al. Evaluation of tomosynthesis elastography in breast-mimicking phantom. Eur J Radiol 2012;81(9):2169–73.

25. Skaane P, Gullien R, Bjorndal H, et al. Digital breast tomosynthesis (DBT): initial experience in a clinical setting. Acta Radiol 2012;53(5):524–9.

26. Fornvik D, Zackrisson S, Ljungberg O, et al. Breast tomosynthesis: accuracy of tumor measurement compared with digital mammography and ultrasonography. Acta Radiol 2010;51(3):240–7.

27. Bernardi D, Ciatto S, Pellegrini M, et al. Prospective study of breast tomosynthesis as a triage to assessment in screening. Breast Cancer Res Treat 2012; 133(1):267–71.

28. Michell MJ, Iqbal A, Wasan RK, et al. A comparison of the accuracy of film-screen mammography, full-field digital mammography, and digital breast tomosynthesis. Clin Radiol 2012;67(10):976–81.

29. Svhan TM, Chakraborty DP, Ikeda D, et al. Breast tomosynthesis and digital mammography: a comparison of diagnostic accuracy. Br J Radiol 2012;85(1019): e1074–82. Available at: http://bjr.birjournals.org/content/early/2012/06/06/bjr. 53282892.full.pdf. Accessed October 17, 2012.
30. Baker JA, Lo JY. Breast tomosynthesis: state-of-the-art and review of the literature. Acad Radiol 2011;18(10):1298–310.
31. Spangler ML, Zuley ML, Sumkin JH, et al. Detection and classification of calcifications on digital breast tomosynthesis and 2D digital mammography: a comparison. AJR Am J Roentgenol 2011;196(2):320–4.
32. Hakim CM, Chough DM, Ganott MA, et al. Digital breast tomosynthesis in the diagnostic environment: a subjective side-by-side review. AJR Am J Roentgenol 2010;195(2):172–6.
33. Helvie MA. Digital mammography imaging: breast tomosynthesis and advanced applications. Radiol Clin North Am 2010;48(5):917–29.
34. Tingberg A. X-ray tomosynthesis: a review of its use for breast and chest imaging. Radiat Prot Dosimetry 2010;139(1–3):100–7.
35. Gennaro G, Toledano A, di Maggio C, et al. Digital breast tomosynthesis versus digital mammography: a clinical performance study. Eur Radiol 2010;20(7): 1545–53.
36. Noroozian M, Hadjiiski L, Rahnama-Moghadam S, et al. Digital breast tomosynthesis is comparable to mammographic spot views for mass characterization. Radiology 2012;262(1):61–8.
37. Orenstein BW. Ultrasound history. Radiology Today 2001;9(24):28.
38. Food and Drug Administration: FDA approves first breast ultrasound imaging system for dense breast tissue. FDA news release, September 18, 2013. Available at: http://www.fda.gov/NewsEvents/Newsroom/PressAnnouncements/ucm319867.htm. Accessed January 7, 2013.
39. Gordon PB. Ultrasound for breast cancer screening and staging. Radiol Clin North Am 2002;40(3):431–41.
40. Kopans D. Breast imaging. 3rd edition. Hagerstown (MD): Lippincott Williams & Wilkins; 2007. p. 82–3.
41. Corsetti V, Houssami N, Ferrari A, et al. Breast screening with ultrasound in women with mammography-negative dense breasts: evidence on incremental cancer detection and false positives, and associated costs. Eur J Cancer 2008;44(4):539–44.
42. Weigert J, Steenbergen S. The Connecticut experiment: the role of ultrasound in the screening of women with dense breasts. Breast J 2012;18(6):517–22.
43. Berg WA, Blume JD, Cormack JB, et al. Combined screening with ultrasound and mammography vs mammography alone in women at elevated risk of breast cancer. JAMA 2008;299(18):2151–63.
44. Ya-jie J, Wei-jun P, Cai C, et al. Application of breast ultrasound in a mammography-based Chinese Breast Screening Study. Cell Biochem Biophys 2013;65(1):37–41.
45. Stomper PC, D'Souza DJ, DiNitto PA, et al. Analysis of parenchymal density on mammograms in 1353 women 25-79 years old. AJR Am J Roentgenol 1996; 167(5):1261–5.
46. Mansour SM, Omar OS. Elastography ultrasound and questionable breast lesions: does it count? Eur J Radiol 2012;81(11):3234–44.
47. Chang JM, Moon WK, Cho N, et al. Clinical application of shear wave elastography (SWE) in the diagnosis of benign and malignant breast diseases. Breast Cancer Res Treat 2011;129(1):89–97.

48. Sadigh F, Carlos RC, Neal CA, et al. Accuracy of quantitative ultrasound elastography for differentiation of malignant and benign breast abnormalities: a meta-analysis. Breast Cancer Res Treat 2012;134(3):923–31.
49. Zhi H, Ou B, Lou BM, et al. Comparison of ultrasound elastography, mammography, and sonography in the diagnosis of solid breast lesions. J Ultrasound Med 2007;26(6):807–15.
50. Cosgrove DO, Berg WA, Dore CJ, et al. Shear wave elastography for breast masses is highly reproducible. Eur Radiol 2012;22(5):1023–32.
51. Barr RG. Sonographic breast elastography: a primer. J Ultrasound Med 2012; 31(5):773–83.
52. Evans A, Whelehan P, Thomson K, et al. Quantitative shear wave ultrasound elastography: initial experience in solid breast masses. Breast Cancer Res 2010;12(6):R104.
53. Chang JM, Moon KW, Cho N, et al. Breast mass evaluation: factors influencing the quality of US elastography. Radiology 2011;259(1):59–64.
54. Gheonea IA, Stoica Z, Bondari S. Differential diagnosis of breast lesions using ultrasound elastography. Indian J Radiol Imaging 2011;21(4):301–5.
55. Garra BS, Cespedes EI, Ophir J, et al. Elastography of breast lesions: initial clinical results. Radiology 1997;202(1):79–86.
56. Berg WA, Cosgrove DO, Dore CJ, et al. Shear-wave elastography improves the specificity of breast US: The BE1 Multinational Study of 939 masses. Radiology 2012;262(2):435–49.
57. Athanasiou A, Tardivon A, Tanter M, et al. Breast lesions: quantitative elastography with supersonic shear imaging-preliminary results. Radiology 2010;256(1): 297–303.
58. Evans A, Whelehan P, Thomson K, et al. Differentiating benign from malignant solid breast masses: value of shear wave elastography according to lesion stiffness combined with greyscale ultrasound according to BI-RADS classification. Br J Cancer 2012;107(2):224–9.
59. Weismann C, Mayr C, Egger H, et al. Breast sonography - 2D, 3D, 4D ultrasound or elastography? Breast Care 2011;6(2):98–103.
60. Itoh A, Ueno E, Tohno E, et al. Breast disease: clinical application of US elastography for diagnosis. Radiology 2006;239(2):341–50.
61. Satake H, Nishio A, Ikeda M, et al. Predictive value for malignancy of suspicious breast masses of BI-RADS categories 4 and 5 using ultrasound elastography and MR diffusion-weighted imaging. AJR Am J Roentgenol 2011;196(1): 202–9.
62. Rzymski P, Skorzewska A, Skibinska-Zielinska M, et al. Factors influencing breast elasticity measured by the ultrasound shear wave elastography-preliminary results. Arch Med Sci 2011;7(1):127–33.
63. Hayashi M, Yamamoto Y, Ibusuki M, et al. Evaluation of tumor stiffness by elastography is predictive for pathologic complete response to neoadjuvant chemotherapy in patients with breast cancer. Ann Surg Oncol 2012;19(9):3042–9.
64. Garra BS. Imaging and estimation of tissue elasticity by ultrasound. Ultrasound Q 2007;23:255–68.
65. Lehman CD, Isaacs C, Schnall MD, et al. Cancer yield of mammography, MR, and US in high-risk women: prospective multi-institution breast cancer screening study. Radiology 2007;244(2):381–8.
66. Kuhl CK, Shrading S, Leutner CC, et al. Mammography, breast ultrasound, and magnetic resonance imaging for surveillance of women at high familial risk for breast cancer. J Clin Oncol 2005;23(33):8469–76.

67. Berg WA, Zhang Z, Lehrer D, et al. Detection of breast cancer with addition of annual screening ultrasound or a single screening MRI to mammography in women with elevated breast cancer risk. JAMA 2012;307(13):1394–404.
68. Plana MN, Carreira C, Muriel A, et al. Magnetic resonance imaging in the preoperative assessment of patients with primary breast cancer: systematic review of diagnostic accuracy and meta-analysis. Eur Radiol 2012;22(1):26–38.
69. Holland R, Veling SH, Mravunac M, et al. Histologic multifocality of Tis, T1-2 breast carcinomas: implications for clinical trials of breast-conserving surgery. Cancer 1985;56(5):979–90.
70. Lehman CD, Gatsonis C, Kuhl CK, et al. MRI evaluation of the contralateral breast in women with recently diagnosed breast cancer. N Engl J Med 2007; 356(13):1295–303.
71. Orel SG, Reynolds C, Schnall MD, et al. Breast carcinoma: MR imaging before re-excisional biopsy. Radiology 1997;205(2):429–36.
72. Yuan Y, Chen XS, Liu SY, et al. Accuracy of MRI in prediction of pathologic complete remission in breast cancer after preoperative therapy: a meta-analysis. AJR Am J Roentgenol 2010;195(1):260–8.
73. Fausto A, Casella D, Mantovani L, et al. Clinical Value of second-look ultrasound: Is there a way to make it objective? Eur J Radiol 2012;81(1):36–40.
74. Makkat S, Luypaert R, Sourbron S, et al. Quantification of perfusion and permeability in breast tumors wlth a deconvolution-based analysis of second-bolus T1-DCE data. J Magn Reson Imaging 2007;25(6):1159–67.
75. Kvistad KA, Rydland J, Vainia J, et al. Breast lesions: evaluation with dynamic contrast-enhanced T1-weighted MR imaging and with T2*-weighted first-pass perfusion MR imaging. Radiology 2000;216(2):545–53.
76. Le Bihan D. Theoretical principles of perfusion imaging: application to magnetic resonance imaging. Invest Radiol 1992;27:6–11.
77. Kawashima M, Katada Y, Shukuya T, et al. MR perfusion imaging using the arterial spin labeling technique for breast cancer. J Magn Reson Imaging 2012; 35(2):436–40.
78. Koo HR, Cho N, Song IC, et al. Correlation of perfusion parameters on dynamic contrast-enhanced MRI with prognostic factors and subtypes of breast cancers. J Magn Reson Imaging 2012;36(1):145–51.
79. deBazelaire C, Calmon R, Thomassin I, et al. Accuracy of perfusion MRI with high spatial but low temporal resolution to assess invasive breast cancer response to neoadjuvant chemotherapy: a retrospective study. BMC Cancer 2011;11:361.
80. Delille JP, Slanetx PJ, Yen ED, et al. Hormone replacement therapy in postmenopausal women: breast tissue perfusion determined with MR imaging-initial observations. Radiology 2005;235(1):36–41.
81. Colditz GA, Hankinson SE, Hunter DJ, et al. The use of estrogens and progestins and the risk of breast cancer in postmenopausal women. N Engl J Med 1995;332(24):1589–93.
82. Biglia N, Mariani L, Sgro L, et al. Increased incidence of lobular breast cancer in women treated with hormone replacement therapy: implications for diagnosis, surgical and medical treatment. Endocr Relat Cancer 2007;14(3):549–67.
83. Chlebowski RT, Anderson GL, Gass M, et al. Estrogen plus progestin and breast cancer incidence and mortality in postmenopausal women. JAMA 2010; 304(15):1684–92.
84. Rossouw JE, Anderson GL, Prentice RL, et al. Risks and benefits of estrogen plus progestin in healthy postmenopausal women principal results from the

Women's Health Initiative Randomized Controlled Trial. JAMA 2002;288(3): 321–33.

85. Zhang B, Zhu B, Li M, et al. Comparative utility of MRI perfusion with MSIDR and DWIBS for the characterization of breast tumors. Acta Radiol 2012;53(6): 607–14.

86. Atuegwu NC, Arlinghaus LR, Li X, et al. Integration of diffusion-weighted MRI data and a simple mathematical model to predict breast tumor cellularity during neoadjuvant chemotherapy. Magn Reson Med 2011;66(6):1689–96.

87. Jensen LR, Garzon B, Heldahl MG, et al. Diffusion-weighted and dynamic contrast-enhanced MRI in evaluation of early treatment effects during neoadjuvant chemotherapy in breast cancer patients. J Magn Reson Imaging 2011; 34(5):1099–109.

88. Kul S, Cansu A, Alhan E, et al. Contribution of diffusion-weighted imaging to dynamic contrast-enhanced MRI in the characterization of breast tumors. AJR Am J Roentgenol 2011;196(1):210–7.

89. Partridge SC, DeMartini WB, Kurland BF, et al. Differential diagnosis of mammographically and clinically occult breast lesions on diffusion-weighted MRI. J Magn Reson Imaging 2010;31(3):562–70.

90. Sharma U, Danishad KK, Seenu V, et al. Longitudinal study of the assessment by MRI and diffusion-weighted imaging of tumor response in patients with locally advanced breast cancer undergoing neoadjuvant chemotherapy. NMR Biomed 2009;22(1):104–13.

91. Sonmez G, Cuce F, Mutlu H, et al. Value of diffusion-weighted MRI in the differentiation of benign and maling breast lesions. CEJMed 2011;123(21–22): 655–61.

92. Yuen S, Yamada K, Goto M, et al. Microperfusion-induced elevation of ADC is suppressed after contrast in breast carcinoma. J Magn Reson Imaging 2009; 29(5):1080–4.

93. Partridge SC, DeMartini WB, Kurland BF, et al. Quantitative diffusion-weighted imaging as an adjunct to conventional breast MRI for improved positive predictive value. AJR Am J Roentgenol 2009;193(6):1716–22.

94. Pereira FP, Martins G, Figueiredo E, et al. Assessment of breast lesions with diffusion-weighted MRI: comparing the use of different b values. AJR Am J Roentgenol 2009;193(4):1030–5.

95. Iacconi C. Diffusion and perfusion of the breast. Eur J Radiol 2010;76(3): 386–90.

96. Partridge SC, Songer L, Sun R, et al. Diffusion-weighted MRI: influence of intravoxel fat signal and breast density on breast tumor conspicuity and apparent diffusion coefficient measurements. Magn Reson Imaging 2011; 29(9):1215–21.

97. Rahbar H, Partridge SC, Eby PR, et al. Characterization of ductal carcinoma in situ on diffusion weighted breast MRI. Eur Radiol 2011;21(9):2011–9.

98. Weigert JM, Bertrand ML, Lanzkowsky L, et al. Results of a multicenter patient registry to determine the clinical impact of breast-specific gamma imaging, a molecular breast imaging technique. AJR Am J Roentgenol 2012;198(1): W69–75.

99. Keto JL, Dirstein L, Sanchez DP, et al. MIRI versus breast-specific gamma imaging (BSGI) in newly diagnosed ductal cell carcinoma-in-situ: a prospective head-to-head trial. Ann Surg Oncol 2012;19(1):249–52.

100. Williams MB, Judy PG, Gunn S, et al. Dual-modality breast tomosynthesis. Radiology 2010;255(1):191–8.

101. Khalkhali I, Baum JK, Villanueva-Meyer J, et al. 99mTc sestamibi breast imaging for the examination of patients with dense and fatty breasts: multicenter study. Radiology 2002;222(1):149–55.

102. O'Connor MD, Li H, Rhodes DJ, et al. Comparison of radiation exposure and associated radiation-induced cancer risks from mammography and molecular imaging of the breast. Med Phys 2010;37(12):6187–98.

103. Tadwalkar RV, Rapelyea JA, Torrente J, et al. Breast-specific gamma imaging as an adjunct modality for the diagnosis of invasive breast cancer with correlation to tumour size and grade. Br J Radiol 2012;85(1014):e212–6.

104. Kim BS, Moon BI, Cha ES. A comparative study of breast-specific gamma imaging with the conventional imaging modality in breast cancer patients with dense breasts. Ann Nucl Med 2012;26(10):823–9.

105. Polan RL, Klein BD, Richman RH. Scintimammography in patients with minimal mammographic of clinical findings. Radiographics 2001;21(3):641–55.

106. Rhodes DJ, Hruska CB, Phillips SW, et al. Dedicated dual-head gamma imaging for breast cancer screening in women with mammographically dense breasts. Radiology 2011;258(1):106–18.

107. Brem RF, Rapelyea JA, Zisman G, et al. Occult breast cancer: scintimammography with high-resolution breast-specific gamma camera in women at high risk for breast cancer. Radiology 2005;237(1):274–80.

108. Khalkhali I, Cutrone JA, Mena IG, et al. Scintimammography: the complementary role of Tc-99m sestamibi prone breast imaging for the diagnosis of breast carcinoma. Radiology 1995;196(2):421–6.

109. Brem RF, Floerke AC, Rapelyea JA, et al. Breast-specific gamma imaging as an adjunct imaging modality for the diagnosis of breast cancer. Radiology 2008; 247(3):651–7.

110. Hendrick RE. Radiation doses and cancer risks from breast imaging studies. Radiology 2010;257(1):246–53.

111. Narayanan D, Madsen KS, Kalonyak JE, et al. Interpretation of positron emission mammography: feature analysis and rates of malignancy. AJR Am J Roentgenol 2011;196(4):956–70.

112. Raylman RR, Majewski S, Smith MF, et al. The positron emission mammography/tomography breast imaging and biopsy system (PEM/PET): design, construction and phantom-based measurements. Phys Med Biol 2008;53(3):637–53.

113. Raylman R, Majewske S, Wojcik R, et al. The potential role of positron emission mammography for detection of breast cancer. A phantom study. Med Phys 2000;27(8):1943–54.

114. Murthy K, Aznar M, Thompson CJ, et al. Results of preliminary clinical trials of the positron emission mammography system PEM-I: a dedicated breast imaging system producing glucose metabolic images using FDG. J Nucl Med 2000;41(11):1851–8.

115. Eo JS, Chun IK, Paeng JC, et al. Imaging sensitivity of dedicated positron emission mammography in relation to tumor size. Breast J 2012;21(1):66–71.

116. MacDonald L, Edwards J, Lewellen T, et al. Clinical imaging characteristics of the positron emission mammography camera: PEM Flex Solo II. J Nucl Med 2009;50(10):1666–75.

117. Shkumat NA, Springer A, Walker CM, et al. Investigating the limit of detectability of a positron emission mammography device: a phantom study. Med Phys 2011; 38(9):5176–85.

118. Wang CL, MacDonald LR, Rogers JV, et al. Positron emission mammography: correlation of estrogen receptor, progesterone receptor, and human epidermal

growth factor receptor 2 status and 18F-FDG. AJR Am J Roentgenol 2011; 197(2):247–55.

119. Levine EZ, Freimanis RI, Perrier ND, et al. Positron emission mammography: initial clinical results. Ann Surg Oncol 2003;10(1):86–91.

120. Schilling K, Narayanan D, Kalinyak JE, et al. Positron emission mammography in breast cancer presurgical planning: comparisons with magnetic resonance imaging. Eur J Nucl Med Mol Imaging 2011;38(1):23–36.

121. Berg WA, Weinberg IN, Narajanan D, et al. High-resolution fluorodeoxyglucose positron emission tomography with compression ("positron emission mammography") is highly accurate in depicting primary breast cancer. Breast J 2006; 12(4):309–23.

122. Kuszyk BS, Corl FM, Franano N, et al. Tumor transport physiology: implication for imaging and imaging-guided therapy. AJR Am J Roentgenol 2001;177(4): 747–53.

123. Weinberg IN, Beylin D, Zavarzin V, et al. Positron emission mammography: high-resolution biochemical breast imaging. Technol Cancer Res Treat 2005;4(1): 55–60.

124. Tafra L, Cheng Z, Uddo J, et al. Pilot clinical trail of 18F-fluorodeoxyglucose positron-emission mammography in the surgical management of breast cancer. Am J Surg 2005;190(4):628–32.

125. Berg WA, Madsen KS, Schilling K, et al. Breast cancer: comparative effectiveness of positron emission mammography and MR imaging in presurgical planning for the ipsilateral breast. Radiology 2011;258(1):59–72.

126. Berg WA, Madsen KS, Schilling K, et al. Comparative effectiveness of positron emission mammography and MRI in the contralateral breast of women with newly diagnosed breast cancer. AJR Am J Roentgenol 2012;198(1):219–32.

127. Springer A, Mawlawi OR. Evaluation of the quantitative accuracy of a commercially available positron emission mammography scanner. Med Phys 2011; 38(4):2132–9.

Benign Breast Disorders

Michaela Onstad, MD, MPH*, Ashley Stuckey, MD

KEYWORDS

- Nipple discharge • Mastalgia • Palpable breast masses
- Adolescent breast disorders • Inflammatory breast conditions

KEY POINTS

- Pathologic nipple discharge is associated with malignancy in 5% to 15% of cases and therefore requires further evaluation.
- Breast pain is common, and in rare instances may be associated with infection or malignancy. Once these are ruled out, mastalgia is a benign condition that can be managed by avoidance of aggravating factors and use of alleviating factors.
- Palpable breast masses should be evaluated by obtaining a history, physical examination, appropriate imaging studies, and biopsy when indicated.
- There are many benign causes that can lead to inflammatory breast lesions; however, breast inflammation may also be a manifestation of malignancy.
- Screening mammograms may reveal benign breast abnormalities that are not otherwise clinically evident or symptomatic. Some require further evaluation and referral to a breast surgeon for surgical excision, whereas others may be associated with an increased risk of developing breast cancer in the future.

INTRODUCTION

Benign lesions of the breast are much more common than malignant lesions, although the actual incidence is difficult to estimate.[1,2] These lesions represent a significant proportion of office visits to the obstetrician-gynecologist, because of either bothersome breast symptoms or abnormal imaging found on screening studies of breast cancer. It is important for the obstetrician-gynecologist to have an understanding of benign breast disease so as to appropriately evaluate and address patients' symptoms, distinguish between benign and malignant processes, determine which benign breast lesions require surgical management, and identify patients who are at increased risk of developing breast cancer.

The authors have nothing to disclose.
Program in Women's Oncology, Department of Obstetrics and Gynecology, Women and Infants Hospital, Warren Alpert Medical School of Brown University, 222 Richmond Street, Providence, RI 02903, USA
* Corresponding author.
E-mail address: maonstad@gmail.com

Obstet Gynecol Clin N Am 40 (2013) 459–473
http://dx.doi.org/10.1016/j.ogc.2013.05.004
0889-8545/13/$ – see front matter © 2013 Elsevier Inc. All rights reserved.

obgyn.theclinics.com

The term benign breast disease encompasses a heterogeneous group of breast lesions. This article reviews common benign breast problems in the manner whereby they are most likely to be presented to the clinician. A discussion of common breast symptoms is followed by a review of benign breast processes found incidentally on imaging and biopsies.

NIPPLE DISCHARGE

As much as 80% of women will experience at least 1 episode of nipple discharge during their reproductive years.[3–5] This discharge can be bothersome to patients, especially if it is copious and persistent, and can also elicit fear, particularly when it is bloody. Most nipple discharge is caused by benign conditions, although up to 15% may have an underlying malignancy[3]; therefore, appropriate evaluation and management is important.

Evaluation should start with obtaining a thorough clinical history. It is important to classify the discharge as unilateral or bilateral, bloody or nonbloody, and spontaneous or provoked. Spontaneous discharge is typically produced in large amounts. It can be found on the patient's clothing and is often readily apparent. Provoked discharge occurs with mechanical stimulation of the duct system, and can usually be reproduced during the physical examination.[6] The history should also include the patient's age, the type and duration of nipple discharge, history of pregnancy and recent parturition, the presence of a palpable breast mass, any history of breast cancer or benign breast conditions, and a thorough review of the patient's current medications.[5] A family history of malignancy, especially breast and ovary, should also be obtained.

Physical examination should include a thorough breast examination to evaluate for any palpable masses. An attempt to reproduce the nipple discharge should also be made, with particular attention paid to determining whether the discharge originates from 1 or multiple ducts of the nipple. Discharge originating from 1 duct is more concerning than flow from multiple ducts. The discharge should be tested for blood, which can easily be done using a Hemoccult card. Other pertinent aspects of the physical examination include evaluation of the eyes for visual field deficits, palpation of the thyroid to evaluate for enlargement or a palpable mass, and evaluation of other secondary signs of pituitary tumor and thyroid abnormalities.[5]

At one time it was recommended that nipple discharge be sampled during examination and sent for cytologic evaluation. Recent studies have suggested that cytology of nipple discharge has poor sensitivity and specificity (16.7% and 66.1%, respectively) and does not add merit to clinical decision making.[7] It is therefore no longer routinely recommended.

Based on the history and physical examination, an attempt should be made to classify the nipple discharge as either physiologic discharge, nonpuerperal galactorrhea, or pathologic discharge (**Box 1**). Physiologic discharge is a benign process. Patients should be reassured that approximately two-thirds of nonlactating women have a small amount of fluid secreted from the nipple with manual expression.[8,9] These women should be advised to avoid frequently checking for nipple discharge, because repeated stimulation of the nipple will promote the production of more discharge. Physiologic discharge often resolves when the nipple is left alone. Nonpuerperal galactorrhea is caused by inappropriately elevated prolactin levels that can be secondary to medications, diseases of the pituitary or thyroid glands, renal failure, or chronic breast stimulation. Because nonpuerperal galactorrhea is not caused by breast abnormality, it is not discussed further in this article. Instead the focus here is on the workup and etiology of pathologic discharge, which is a symptom of a

---

Box 1
Classification of nipple discharge

Physiologic Discharge

   Various colors (yellow, white, green, brown, blue-black)

   Does not occur spontaneously

   Originates from multiple ducts

Nonpuerperal Galactorrhea

   Milk production unrelated to pregnancy or nursing, or occurring more than 1 year after nursing

   Spontaneous or provoked

   Typically persistent

   Occasionally voluminous

   Associated with chronic breast stimulation and hyperprolactinemia

Pathologic Discharge

   Spontaneous

   Unilateral

   Typically arises from a single duct opening

   Bloody, serous, serosanguinous, or watery

   Persistent

---

pathologic process within the breast. Malignancy is found in 5% to 15% of patients with pathologic nipple discharge.[8]

Evaluation of Pathologic Discharge

All pathologic discharge should undergo further evaluation, which should begin with imaging studies to determine whether there is an identifiable mass or abnormality associated with the discharge. A mammogram and/or ultrasonogram should be ordered as initial steps, with biopsy performed when indicated.[5,6,8,10] The use of additional imaging studies, such as diagnostic ductography and magnetic resonance imaging (MRI) of the breast, is controversial.[8,10]

Diagnostic ductography involves the installation of contrast material into the duct that has been identified as producing the nipple discharge. This procedure reportedly is a technically challenging one, and requires that the duct is able to be cannulated. Morrogh and colleagues[10] describe a series of 178 patients with pathologic nipple discharge who underwent ductography, 76% of whom had an otherwise negative evaluation with breast examination, mammogram, and ultrasonogram. Cannulation was successful in 84% of patients. In this series, ductography had sensitivity of 76% for detecting malignancy, specificity of 11%, and a positive predictive value of 11%. A patient with a negative ductogram (and negative mammogram and ultrasonogram), therefore, may still harbor a malignancy, and requires surgical management. Some breast surgeons are of the opinion that, despite this, ductography can be useful in identifying the location of the lesion to aid in minimizing the amount of tissue removed during surgery.[8]

The use of breast MRI for evaluation of nipple discharge is also controversial. Lorenzon and colleagues[11] retrospectively evaluated 38 women with pathologic nipple discharge who underwent mammography, ultrasonography, and breast MRI before surgery. Breast MRI had a sensitivity of 94.7% for detecting malignancy and specificity of 78.9%. Three of 5 cancers that were present in this study were detected by MRI alone. The investigators concluded that MRI should be ordered in all patients with pathologic nipple discharge who have a negative mammogram and ultrasonogram. Opponents of this strategy argue that MRI carries a significant false-positive rate and is costly, and that there is limited availability of MR-guided biopsies at many centers in the United States.

At present, ultimately all pathologic nipple discharge requires a tissue diagnosis to appropriately evaluate for malignancy. When an abnormality is detected by a mammogram or ultrasonogram, an image-guided biopsy should be performed. In the setting of a normal mammogram and ultrasonogram, surgical excision should be performed, requiring referral to a breast surgeon. When a specific duct can be identified on examination, a selective duct excision can be performed to obtain a tissue diagnosis. Otherwise, a central duct excision is recommended.[12]

Papillary Lesions

Papillary lesions of the breast represent a spectrum of pathology that includes benign, atypical, and malignant lesions. Papillary lesions are more common among women between the ages of 30 and 50 years.[8] When papillary lesions are located near the nipple, they typically present with pathologic bloody nipple discharge. However, these lesions may also be detected by abnormal imaging studies or may be found incidentally on biopsy performed for other indications.

Intraductal papillomas are benign tumors of the epithelium of mammary ducts. Approximately 50% are single lesions.[8] These tumors can range in size from less than 3 mm up to several centimeters. Grossly they are tan or pink, tend to be friable, and are typically associated with a dilated duct. Microscopically they consist of multiple branching papillae with a fibrovascular core lined by epithelium. Surgical excision of these lesions is recommended and is generally curative.

Atypical papillomas are papillomas with atypical features found in the epithelial cells. These tumors carry an increased risk of being associated with in situ and invasive breast cancers, and should be surgically excised when diagnosed by core biopsy.[13]

Papillomatosis describes papillomas containing ductal hyperplasia without atypia (proliferation of the ductal epithelial cells). Juvenile papillomatosis is a disease described in women younger than 30 years. It typically presents as a localized mass and microscopically involves ductal hyperplasia without atypia, and may also be associated with other benign proliferative findings.[13] Approximately 10% of patients with juvenile papillomatosis have breast cancer.

Papillary carcinoma, mentioned for the sake of completeness, is more commonly found among women older than 60 years.

Mammary Duct Ectasia

Mammary duct ectasia is characterized by dilation of the mammary ducts. If symptomatic it typically causes nipple discharge, which is frequently bilateral, present in multiple ducts, and of various colors (not typically pathologic discharge). The discharge may be described as cheesy or viscous.[8] It occurs most often in the perimenopausal period, but has also been described among younger women, children, and men.[14] The cause is unknown, but an association with smoking has been described.[15] Mammary duct ectasia generally does not require surgery and should be managed conservatively. When asymptomatic, duct ectasia does not require treatment. Duct excision is recommended if the clinical presentation and mammographic findings are otherwise suggestive of malignancy.[8]

BREAST PAIN

Many women will experience breast pain at some point in their lives. Most of the time this pain is self-limited and resolves on its own; however, for some women the pain can be persistent. In a questionnaire sent to women in South Wales, 66% of respondents reported having some breast pain and 21% reported having severe breast pain. Less than half of the women with severe breast pain had discussed it with their physician.[16] Nonetheless, breast pain is one of the most common breast symptoms encountered by primary care physicians.[17] In rare instances, breast pain may be related to infection, malignancy, or a condition not associated with the breast. **Box 2** lists the extramammary causes that can present as breast pain. Once these possibilities are ruled out, mastalgia is a benign entity.

Evaluation of breast pain should begin with a detailed history and physical examination. The history should help to classify the pain as cyclical or noncyclical, explore for potential aggravating and alleviating factors, and evaluate for extramammary causes. **Box 3** lists important aspects to include in the history.[6,18]

The physical examination should involve careful observation and palpation of the affected area, which can be reassuring to the patient and indicates that her fears and concerns are being taken seriously.[6] In observing the patient, take note of skin marks along the bra line (indicating an ill-fitting bra) or shoulder marks from heavy handbag shoulder straps. Evaluate for any other skin lesions, including lesions characteristic of herpes zoster. Perform a thorough breast examination in the sitting and supine positions, evaluating for masses or abnormalities. To isolate pain related to the chest wall (chostochondritis) and differentiate it from true mastalgia, have the patient lay on her side or in the sitting position, leaning forward, allowing the breast tissue to be displaced before palpating the underlying chest wall.

A mammogram and/or breast ultrasonography should be ordered as indicated for any abnormalities discovered on examination. Whether a diagnostic mammogram should be ordered to further evaluate mastalgia in a woman with a normal breast examination is controversial. A study by Dujim and colleagues[19] concludes that in women with mastalgia alone, mammography provides reassurance. Others believe that mammography is widely overused in this setting.[17] It would certainly be appropriate

---

Box 2
Extramammary causes that may present as breast pain

Costochondritis

Tietze syndrome

Cervical radiculopathy

Myocardial ischemia

Pneumonia

Irritation of the pleura

Esophageal spasm

Rib fracture

Shingles

Box 3
Obtaining a clinical history of breast pain

Location

Unilateral versus bilateral

Localized within a specific area of the breast

Deep or superficial

Involving chest wall

Timing

Constant versus variable

Variations with menstrual cycle

Associated symptoms

Symptoms of infection (fever, chills, erythema, swelling)

Symptoms of malignancy (palpable mass, nipple retraction, skin changes)

Previous surgery

Recent injury

Aggravating and alleviating factors

Caffeine use

Tobacco use

Nonsteroidal anti-inflammatory use

Severity

Recent weight changes

Loss or gain of more than 10 lb (4.5 kg) in past year

Medications

Hormonal medications

Antidepressants

Spironolactone

Methyldopa

---

to order a screening mammogram for women older than 40 if not performed in the past year.

Cyclical Breast Pain

Approximately two-thirds of women with breast pain have cyclical pain.[20] By definition, cyclical pain occurs in a predictable pattern with the menstrual cycle. It is typically worse in the luteal phase and is relieved by the onset of menses. It is frequently bilateral, and is often most severe in the upper outer quadrants. Cyclical pain is most common among women in the reproductive years, and typically improves after menopause.

The etiology of cyclical breast pain (mastalgia) is poorly understood. Many patients with cyclical mastalgia also have breast nodularity and tenderness. However, there is no consistent association between symptoms and breast histology,[17] and fibrocystic changes are now thought to be secondary to normal physiologic breast involution as opposed to a disease process.[21] Cyclical breast pain is likely due to hormonal changes, given that it occurs during the reproductive years and fluctuates with the menstrual cycle. However, studies have demonstrated that women with cyclical mastalgia have hormone levels similar to those of women who do not have breast pain. It has been suggested that, rather than differences in absolute hormone levels, an increased sensitivity to hormones may explain cyclical mastalgia.[17]

Management of cyclical mastalgia should start with reassurance. Women are often relieved that breast pain is common and is rarely the sole manifestation of breast cancer.[6] For some women, no further treatment is needed. In addition, there are lifestyle and dietary interventions that may alleviate cyclic mastalgia. The use of a well-fitting support bra and initiation of regular exercise have been proved to improve mastalgia.[6,17,22] The elimination of caffeine (and other methylxanthines) is more controversial, as it has been shown to reduce the severity of mastalgia in some studies but has proved to be ineffective in other studies.[17] Avoiding caffeine is still commonly recommended because it carries few risks and may have other health benefits. Vitamin E supplementation also may be effective in decreasing pain; however, this has not yet been confirmed by a placebo-controlled trial. Evening primrose oil has been demonstrated to reduce mastalgia in placebo-controlled trials, although it often takes a long course of treatment (at least 4 months) to achieve this result.[17]

Endocrine therapies (such as bromocriptine, danazol, and tamoxifen) have been shown to be effective in treating cyclical mastalgia; however, such treatments are associated with side effects that limit their use.[17] In a meta-analysis evaluating randomized controlled trials for the treatment of cyclical mastalgia by Srivastava and colleagues,[23] bromocriptine, danazol, and tamoxifen were all found to offer significant relief from mastalgia. High-quality data comparing each of these medications with one another are not yet available.

Noncyclical Breast Pain

Noncyclical breast pain does not follow the typical menstrual pattern. It is more likely to be unilateral and to vary in location. It is important to evaluate for specific pathologic processes that can be treated, such as trauma and postoperative pain syndromes, breast cysts, duct ectasia, and periductal mastitis.

Trauma to the breast and breast surgery can obviously cause pain in the acute setting and is typically clinically obvious. What may be less obvious is that a prior history of trauma to the breast and previous surgery may lead to fat necrosis or other remodeling processes, causing pain that can persist for many years after the initial event.[6] Imaging studies of fat necrosis are often concerning for malignancy and should be evaluated by tissue biopsy, even when a patient gives a history of prior trauma to the region.[24] Mondor disease is a form of superficial thrombophlebitis of the anterior thoracoabdominal wall that can be caused by trauma (including muscular strain and electrocution) or surgery. It presents with a subcutaneous, tender, cord-like induration between the epigastric and axillary regions. The diagnosis is confirmed by ultrasonography, and treatment involves anti-inflammatory medications.[25]

Large palpable breast cysts can be associated with breast pain. These cysts can be confirmed by ultrasonography and are typically effectively treated by needle aspiration. Simple breast cysts are typically benign in nature. However, if a bloody aspirate is obtained, a mass persists after aspiration, or the cyst recurs, a biopsy should be performed.[6]

Periductal mastitis is another important cause of noncyclical mastalgia. Examination may demonstrate overlying skin erythema, a subareolar breast mass or abscess, or a fistula. Diagnosis can be confirmed by ultrasonography. Surgical treatment is usually indicated (see later discussion).

PALPABLE BREAST MASSES

A palpable breast mass may be described by the patient as a finding she noticed on her own, or may be discovered on routine physical examination. A medical history should be obtained, including the length of time the mass has been present, changes in size over time, fluctuations with the menstrual cycle, and any associated pain, skin changes, or nipple discharge.[26] Prior history of breast health should be obtained, including past breast biopsies or surgery and any episodes of abnormal imaging. Risk factors for breast cancer should be assessed, including a detailed family history.[6]

A clinical breast examination should be performed with visual inspection, palpation of the axillae, supraclavicular, and cervical lymph node regions, and palpation of bilateral breasts.[27] Any palpable finding should be described using clear, descriptive terminology, including the size, tissue consistency, mobility, margin characteristics, distance from the areolar edge, and the clock-face position. Occasionally a patient may present for evaluation of a breast mass, but during the clinical examination neither she nor the provider is unable to palpate it. In this instance it is recommended that she return for a repeat breast examination in 2 to 3 months, possibly in the follicular phase of the menstrual cycle.[27]

When a dominant mass or concerning area is identified on examination, imaging studies should be obtained. The ordering physician should describe the exact location (including clock-face position and distance from the nipple or areolar margin) to ensure that these studies target the area of interest. Breast ultrasonography should be performed to determine whether the lesion is solid or cystic and to further characterize it as suspicious or benign-appearing. For women older than 30 years, a diagnostic mammogram should also be ordered.[27] Mammography can help determine whether a lesion is potentially malignant, and also screens for occult disease in surrounding tissue. The results of these imaging studies should be reported by the radiologist using the Breast Imaging Reporting and Data System (BI-RADS), which classifies studies according to the level of suspicion for malignancy (further discussed in the article by Garcia and colleagues elsewhere in this issue).

In some instances, mammography and ultrasonography cannot identify any lesion that correlates with the palpable findings. If the palpable area persists and remains concerning, a biopsy or referral to a breast surgeon should be obtained. A small percentage of breast cancers are present only as a palpable mass but cannot be identified with imaging studies, so it is important to consider that normal imaging studies cannot completely exclude malignancy.[18]

Imaging may suggest a specific benign lesion based on its characteristic appearance (BI-RADS 2) or may suggest that the lesion is "probably benign" (BI-RADS 3). If the patient's history and physical examination are also consistent with benign disease, the lesion can be followed clinically or with short-interval follow-up. If the clinical findings remain worrisome despite reassuring imaging, a biopsy of the lesion is recommended for further evaluation.[27] Imaging studies that result as BI-RADS 4 or 5 are more suspicious for malignancy, and a tissue biopsy is warranted.

Percutaneous core-needle biopsy is now the most commonly used and favored modality for obtaining a breast-tissue specimen for diagnosis.[8] It is a minimally invasive technique, has few complications, and minimizes surgical changes to the breast.[27] Fine-needle aspiration was used more commonly in the past, but has been criticized for having a relatively high rate of obtaining samples deemed inadequate or suboptimal. One study found 28% of samples inadequate and an additional 22% less than optimal.[28] When the pretest probability of malignancy is low, fine-needle aspiration can be used in combination with clinical examination and imaging studies, which is termed the triple test. When all 3 studies suggest a benign process, there is a 99% certainty that the mass is benign.[27] Surgical excisional biopsy is generally reserved for special circumstances when core-needle biopsy cannot be performed, or when the results of the core-needle biopsy require that additional tissue be obtained to confirm a benign diagnosis.[27]

Fibroadenoma

Fibroadenomas are common benign lesions of the breast that arise from the epithelium and stroma of the terminal duct–lobular unit.[8] These lesions are most common in young women between the ages of 20 and 40 years, but can be found in women of any age. Fibroadenomas typically present as a discrete painless breast mass discovered by the patient. On examination a fibroadenoma is smooth, mobile, well circumscribed, and has a rubbery consistency. Approximately 10% to 20% are multiple and bilateral.[8] On ultrasonography they are typically elliptical or lobulated, and are "wider than tall." Most measure less than 3 cm in size. A fibroadenoma larger than 6 cm is referred to as a giant fibroadenoma, and must be distinguished from a phyllodes tumor (see later discussion). Unlike fibroadenoma, phyllodes tumors may enlarge quickly and can visibly distort the breast.[18]

A fibroadenoma that has been confirmed by core-needle biopsy does not require surgical excision unless it is bothersome to the patient or clinically enlarges over time.[18] Newer technologies, such as ultrasound-guided vacuum-assisted removal and cryoablation, offer minimally invasive approaches to treating small fibroadenomas smaller than 2 cm.[8]

Phyllodes Tumor

Phyllodes tumors are rare, accounting for less than 1% of all breast tumors.[29] These tumors are fibroepithelial, with the potential to become malignant, recur, and metastasize to other organs.[8] Most women present with a firm palpable mass with examination findings similar to those of fibroadenoma. The average size is 4 to 5 cm, but they can be small (1 cm) or extremely large (>30 cm). Unfortunately, there are no specific imaging features on mammography, ultrasonography, or MRI that can distinguish a phyllodes tumor from a fibroadenoma.[29]

Histologically, phyllodes tumors are classified as benign, borderline, or malignant. Of note, even benign phyllodes tumors recur, and both borderline and malignant tumors have the ability to metastasize. Management of nonmetastatic phyllodes tumors requires wide local excision with margins 1 cm or greater. Total mastectomy is recommended if negative margins cannot be obtained.[29]

Hamartoma

Hamartomas account for 4.8% of benign breast tumors,[8] and consist of ducts, lobules, fibrous stroma, and adipose tissue all arranged in a disorganized fashion. Hamartomas present as painless, well-circumscribed, mobile masses, and are most common among women aged 30 to 50 years. On ultrasonography they appear as a solid mass. Mammography demonstrates a sharply defined, homogeneously dense mass.[30] Once confirmed by tissue biopsy, if no atypia is identified they can be managed with observation alone.[8]

Fibromatosis

Also referred to as a desmoid tumor, fibromatosis of the breast is similar to fibromatosis at other sites. It is an uncommon tumor characterized as an infiltrating, well-differentiated proliferation of spindle cells.[8] Fibromatosis may be seen in patients with a history of familial adenomatous polyposis (FAP). Women present with a palpable mass that may adhere to the chest wall or cause dimpling or retraction of the skin. For this reason, it can be suspicious of malignancy.[31] On ultrasonography, it can appear lobulated or spiculated, with irregular margins.[32] It is frequently not detectable on mammography, but may appear spiculated and irregular when seen.[32] MRI is the best method for determining the size and extent of the lesion.[31] The recommended treatment is wide local excision. Positive margins are associated with a high risk of recurrence, and should be re-excised.[8]

Lactating Adenoma

The most common palpable breast mass among young pregnant women is a lactating adenoma,[33] which only arise during pregnancy and in the postpartum period. Women present with well-circumscribed masses that typically measure 2 to 4 cm.[8] Ultrasonography demonstrates an ovoid mass with well-defined margins. A core-needle biopsy should be performed to obtain a diagnosis and evaluate for malignancy. Histologically a lactating adenoma appears as a lobulated mass of enlarged acini surrounded by a basement membrane and edematous stroma.[34] Approximately 5% of cases are complicated by hemorrhage and infarction of the breast tissue. It is thought that infarction occurs because of relative vascular insufficiency of the breast during this time, owing to a high requirement for blood supply during pregnancy and lactation.[34] Following completion of pregnancy and lactation, lactating adenomas typically involute. If the mass persists or enlarges, surgical excision should be considered.[34]

ADOLESCENT BREAST DISORDERS

Breast concerns among adolescent women are common. Concerns about nipple discharge and breast pain may arise in this age group. The evaluation and management of these problems in adolescents is similar to that conducted for adults. Adolescent women can be given greater reassurance than their older counterparts that the incidence of breast cancer among women of their age is very rare. Nonetheless, their concerns should be adequately evaluated and addressed.

The most common breast masses among adolescent women are fibroadenomas. Giant fibroadenomas and phyllodes tumors can also occur, and should be considered in the differential diagnosis. Palpable masses should be evaluated with ultrasonography. There is no role for mammography in the adolescent woman.

A few additional concerns that may arise in adolescence are covered here, including breast asymmetry, tuberous breasts, and juvenile hypertrophy.

Breast Asymmetry

During puberty, it is not uncommon for one breast to develop more rapidly than the other. On physical examination, asymmetry is noted without any palpable masses. Ultrasonography may be ordered for further evaluation of a mass contributing to asymmetry when warranted. With a negative evaluation, patients and their parents can be reassured that asymmetry often becomes less noticeable with age. When plastic-surgery procedures are desired, they should be delayed until after full breast development is complete.[35]

Tuberous Breast Deformity

Tuberous breasts are breasts with a limited breast base and overdeveloped nipple-areolar complex. This condition may be caused by the use of exogenous steroids or hormones. When extreme, they can be surgically managed.[35]

Juvenile Hypertrophy

Juvenile hypertrophy describes extreme macromastia with pathologic overgrowth of bilateral breasts, with onset at menarche. Each breast may weigh as much as 30 to 50 lb (13.6–22.7 kg), leading to back and neck strain. Surgical management with reduction mammoplasty is often considered in the older teen or young adult.[35]

INFLAMMATORY LESIONS

There are many benign causes that can lead to inflammatory breast lesions; however, breast inflammation may also be a manifestation of malignancy. It is important to appropriately evaluate these lesions, prevent complications of infectious causes, and accurately and promptly diagnose inflammatory breast cancer. This section discusses benign inflammatory lesions, ways to distinguish them from malignant lesions, and the management of such lesions. Inflammatory lesions may be classified as infectious, noninfectious, and malignant.

The evaluation should begin with a thorough history. The patient should describe the timing of the redness and whether the extent of redness has changed over time. Any associated masses should be noted as well as systemic symptoms including fevers, chills, and weight loss. Special attention should be paid to risk factors for breast infections such as lactation, smoking, prior infections or abscesses, nipple piercing, and recent surgery.[36] Physical examination should focus on the breast and axilla, evaluating for erythema, masses, purulent drainage, and lymphadenopathy. Imaging studies such as ultrasonography and/or mammography may be indicated to evaluate for associated masses or evidence of malignancy.

Lactational Infections

Lactational mastitis is the most common form of mastitis. It occurs in approximately 2% to 10% of breastfeeding women and typically occurs during the first 6 weeks of breastfeeding or weaning.[8] Lactational mastitis is associated with engorgement, poor milk drainage, and excoriated nipples. Women may present with fevers, malaise, and occasionally rigors. On examination there is typically erythema, localized engorgement, or swelling. Treatment consists of antibiotics and encouragement of milk flow from the engorged segment.[37] A smaller proportion of breastfeeding women (0.4%) develop a breast abscess, which in some cases may be due to suboptimal management of mastitis.[37]

A suspected breast abscess or any mastitis that does not resolve despite the completion of a course of antibiotics should be evaluated with ultrasonography. When an abscess is identified, management should include either aspiration of the fluid or incision and drainage. When the tissue overlying the abscess is normal, aspiration may be the most suitable option. Aspiration should be done in combination with the use of oral antibiotics, and reaspiration should be performed every 2 to 3 days until no further purulent fluid can be drained.[37] If, however, the skin overlying the abscess appears thinned or necrotic, it may be more advisable to proceed to incision and drainage rather than attempt to manage with aspiration, given that these patients have a higher likelihood of failing treatment with repeated aspiration.[37]

Nonlactational Infections

Nonlactational infections include periductal mastitis, granulomatous lobular mastitis, and skin-associated infections (such as infected epidermal cysts and cellulitis of the breast). Periductal mastitis describes a condition of damaged subareolar ducts that become infected. Smoking tobacco is considered to be a major causative factor, with 90% of patients who develop periductal mastitis being smokers.[37] Women with diabetes are more likely to have recurrent infections.[37] Granulomatous lobular mastitis is less common, and typically presents as a peripheral inflammatory mass of unknown cause. Nonlactating abscesses can be managed similarly to lactating abscesses, with aspiration or incision and drainage combined with oral antibiotics. Recurrent infections are more common than they are among lactating abscesses, typically because the underlying abnormality in the central ducts persists. Women who have recurrent disease may require definitive surgery with total duct excision, which removes the diseased ducts to prevent infection from recurring.[37]

Malignant Inflammatory Lesions

Inflammatory breast cancer mimics an infectious process. Most patients who are diagnosed with inflammatory breast cancer were initially misdiagnosed as having an infectious process. When inflammation does not resolve with treatment, inflammatory breast cancer should be considered. A mammogram and ultrasonogram should be ordered, and any suspicious findings should be biopsied. The skin can also be biopsied to confirm the diagnosis.[15]

BENIGN BREAST ABNORMALITY DETECTED ON IMAGING AND BIOPSY

Routine screening mammograms may reveal benign breast abnormalities that are not otherwise clinically evident or symptomatic. On imaging, they may appear similar to malignancies: as calcifications, a mass or density, asymmetry, or an area of architectural distortion.[18] Of all screening mammograms performed, approximately 10% will require additional imaging. Of those, approximately 8% to 10% will require biopsy. Breast cancer will be detected in 4 of every 1000 women undergoing screening mammography. The remaining women who undergo biopsy for abnormal imaging findings will be diagnosed with benign breast disease.[38,39] It is important for the obstetrician-gynecologist to be familiar with these diseases. Some require further evaluation and referral to a breast surgeon for surgical excision. Others may be associated with an increased risk of developing breast cancer in the future. In general, these lesions can be classified as nonproliferative lesions, proliferative lesions without atypia, and proliferative lesions with atypia.

Nonproliferative Lesions

Breast cysts are common nonproliferative lesions found incidentally on imaging, which originate from the terminal ductal lobule unit and can vary in size from microscopic to large, clinically palpable masses. Small simple breast cysts found incidentally on imaging are nearly always benign and do not require any further workup. Other nonproliferative lesions include mild hyperplasia and papillary apocrine change (commonly found in fibrocystic disease), which also do not require any further workup. In general, nonproliferative lesions are not considered to increase a woman's risk of developing breast cancer.[27]

Proliferative Lesions Without Atypia

Proliferative lesions without atypia include fibroadenomas, intraductal papillomas without atypia, sclerosing adenosis or radial scar, and pseudoangiomatous stromal hyperplasia (PASH). Fibroadenomas and papillomas are described in an earlier section of this article. A radial scar is a complex sclerosing lesion with a radial center. When seen on a mammogram it appears spiculated, similar to a small invasive carcinoma. Histologically, it consists of proliferative changes surrounding a fibroelastic core that can mimic the appearance of a malignancy. When diagnosed on a core biopsy, an excisional biopsy is generally recommended to evaluate the entirety of the lesion. Sclerosing adenosis can also present as a suspicious finding on imaging, but the risk of subsequent breast cancer is small, and no treatment is required.

PASH is a myofibroblastic proliferation of the breast. On mammography it appears as an oval mass without microcalcifications. When PASH is diagnosed by percutaneous core biopsy, no further management is necessary as long as the abnormality is concordant with the imaging findings. If imaging is otherwise suspicious, surgical excision is recommended.[40] There is no increased risk of developing subsequent breast cancer.[40]

Proliferative Lesions with Atypia

Proliferative lesions with atypia include various types of epithelial hyperplasia with atypical cells. Women diagnosed with these lesions carry an increased risk of developing breast cancer, with a relative risk of 3.9 to 13.0.[15] Depending on the type of cells involved, they are classified as atypical ductal hyperplasia, atypical lobular hyperplasia, or flat epithelial hyperplasia. When diagnosed on core biopsy, these lesions should undergo surgical excision because a significant number are "upgraded" to carcinoma in situ on excision.[8]

Given that women with these benign lesions are identified as having an increased risk of breast cancer, they can be counseled about options for increased screening and risk reduction, as discussed in the article by Green elsewhere in this issue.

SUMMARY

Benign breast lesions are much more common than malignant lesions. Women may present with specific complaints related to their breasts, or may have abnormal screening mammograms that lead to the diagnosis of benign breast disease. Evaluation should include obtaining a relevant history, performing a physical examination, ordering imaging studies as appropriate, and obtaining a tissue diagnosis when indicated. Some benign breast diseases have been associated with an increased risk for developing breast cancer.

REFERENCES

1. Cole P, Mark Elwood J, Kaplan SD. Incidence rates and risk factors of benign breast neoplasms. Am J Epidemiol 1978;108:112–20.
2. Bartow SA, Pathak DR, Black WC, et al. Prevalence of benign, atypical, and malignant breast lesions in populations at different risk for breast cancer. A forensic autopsy study. Cancer 1987;60:2751–60.
3. Hughes LE, Mansel RE, Webster DJ, et al. Benign disorders and diseases of the breast. London: WB Saunders; 2000.
4. Issacs JH. Other nipple discharge. Clin Obstet Gynecol 1994;37:898–902.

5. Hussain AN, Policarpio C, Vincent MT. Evaluating nipple discharge. Obstet Gynecol Surv 2006;61:278–83.

6. Marchant DJ. Breast disease. Philadelphia: WB Saunders; 1997.

7. Kooistra BW, Wauters C, van de Ven S, et al. The diagnostic evaluation of nipple discharge cytology in 618 consecutive patients. Eur J Surg Oncol 2009;35(6): 573.

8. Kuerer HM. Kuerer's breast surgical oncology. New York: McGraw-Hill; 2010.

9. Falkenberry SS. Nipple discharge. Obstet Gynecol Clin North Am 2002;29:21–9.

10. Morrogh M, Park A, Elkin EB, et al. Lessons learned from 416 cases of nipple discharge of the breast. Am J Surg 2010;200:73–80.

11. Lorenzon M, Zuiani C, Linda A, et al. Magnetic resonance imaging in patients with nipple discharge: should we recommend it? Eur Radiol 2011;21:899–907.

12. Vargas HI, Romero L, Chlebowski RT. Management of bloody nipple discharge. Curr Treat Options Oncol 2002;3:157–61.

13. Ibarra JA. Papillary lesions of the breast. Breast J 2006;12(3):237–51.

14. Rahal S. Mammary duct ectasia: an overview. Breast J 2011;6:694–5.

15. Guray M, Sahin AA. Benign breast diseases: classification, diagnosis, and management. Oncologist 2006;11:435–49.

16. Maddox P, Mansel R. Management of breast pain and nodularity. World J Surg 1989;13:699–705.

17. Millet AV, Dirbas FM. Clinical management of breast pain: a review. Obstet Gynecol Surv 2002;57(7):451–61.

18. Miltenburg DM, Speights VO. Benign breast disease. Obstet Gynecol Clin North Am 2008;35:285–300.

19. Dujim LE, Guilt GL, Hendriks JH. Value of breast imaging in women with painful breasts: observational follow-up study. BMJ 1998;317:1492–5.

20. Davies EL, Gateley CA, Miers M, et al. The long-term course of mastalgia. J R Soc Med 1998;91(9):462.

21. Jorgensen J, Watt BS. Cyclical mastalgia and breast pathology. Acta Chir Scand 1985;151:319–21.

22. Hadi MS. Sports brassier: is it a solution for mastalgia? Breast J 2000;6:407–9.

23. Srivastava A, Mansel RE, Arvind N, et al. Evidence-based management of mastalgia: a meta-analysis of randomized trials. Breast 2007;16:503–12.

24. Tan PH, Lai LM, Carrington EV, et al. Fat necrosis of the breast—a review. Breast 2006;15:313–8.

25. Alvarez-Garrido H, Garrido-Rios AA, Sanz-Munoz C, et al. Mondor's disease. Clin Exp Dermatol 2009;34:753–6.

26. Klein S. Evaluation of palpable breast masses. Am Fam Physician 2005;71(9): 1731–8.

27. Pearlman MD, Griffin JL. Benign breast disease. Obstet Gynecol 2010;116(3): 747–58.

28. Saxe A, Phillips E, Orfanou P, et al. Role of sample adequacy in fine needle aspiration biopsy of palpable breast lesions. Am J Surg 2001;182:369–71.

29. Khosravi-Shahi P. Management of non metastatic phyllodes tumors of the breast: review of the literature. Surg Oncol 2011;20:e143–8.

30. Tovar JR, Reguero Callejas ME, Alaez Chillaron AB, et al. Mammary hamartoma. Clin Transl Oncol 2006;8(4):290–3.

31. Schwartz GS, Drotman M, Rosenblatt R, et al. Fibromatosis of the breast: case report and current concepts in the management of an uncommon lesion. Breast J 2006;12(1):66–71.

32. Taylor TV, Sosa J. Bilateral breast fibromatosis: case report and review of the literature. J Surg Educ 2011;68(4):320–5.
33. Collins JC, Liao S, Wile AG. Surgical management of breast masses in pregnant women. J Reprod Med 1996;40:785–8.
34. Baker TP, Lenert JF, Parker J, et al. Lactating adenoma: a diagnosis of exclusion. Breast J 2001;7(5):354–7.
35. Arca MJ, Caniano DA. Breast disorders in the adolescent patient. Adolesc Med 2004;15:473–85.
36. Froman J, Landercasper J, Ellis R, et al. Red breast as a presenting complaint at a breast center: an institutional review. Surgery 2011;149(6):813–9.
37. Dixon JM, Khan LR. Treatment of breast infection. BMJ 2011;342:d396.
38. Neal L, Tortorelli CL, Nassar A. Clinician's guide to imaging and pathologic findings in benign breast disease. Mayo Clin Proc 2010;85(3):274–9.
39. Jaunoo SS, Thrush S, Dunn P. Pseudoangiomatous stromal hyperplasia (PASH): a brief review. Int J Surg 2011;9:20–2.
40. Hargarden GC, Yeh ED, Georgian-Smith D, et al. Analysis of the mammographic and sonographic features of pseudoangiomatous stromal hyperplasia. AJR Am J Roentgenol 2008;191(2):359–63.

Hereditary Breast/Ovarian Cancer Syndrome

A Primer for Obstetricians/Gynecologists

Dana Meaney-Delman, MD, MPH*, Cecelia A. Bellcross, PhD, MS

KEYWORDS

- BRCA1 • BRCA2 • Hereditary breast cancer • Hereditary ovarian cancer
- Genetic testing • Clinical management

KEY POINTS

- Families with hereditary breast and ovarian cancer (HBOC) syndrome are at substantially greater risk for breast and ovarian cancer than the general population.
- Genetic cancer risk assessment is important to identify high-risk families.
- Effective, evidence-based preventive strategies are available to reduce the risk of cancer and overall morbidity and mortality.
- Women's health providers knowledgeable about HBOC can greatly improve the lives of HBOC families.

INTRODUCTION

Breast cancer remains the most common female cancer, affecting approximately 1 in 8 women over the course of their lifetime.[1] Of the more than 200,000 of breast cancers that occur in the United States each year, most are considered sporadic, 15% to 20% are familial, and 5% to 10% are hereditary.[1–3] **Table 1** shows the general distinctions between these three classifications of genetic risk for breast cancer. Ovarian cancer affects fewer women over the course of their lifetimes (1 in 70), but it remains associated with late detection and high mortality, and 20% to 25% of epithelial ovarian cancers may have a hereditary cause.[1,4]

Hereditary cancers are associated with inherited, primarily dominant, mutations in cancer-predisposing genes, including tumor suppressor, DNA mismatch repair, and oncogenes. The cancers are characterized by early age of onset, multifocal or bilateral disease, and high penetrance, with lifetime risks typically 5-fold to 10-fold that of the general population. Hereditary breast/ovarian cancer syndrome (HBOC) accounts for

Disclosures: The authors have nothing to disclose.
Department of Gynecology and Obstetrics, Emory University School of Medicine, 49 Jesse Hill Jr Drive, Atlanta, GA 30303, USA
* Corresponding author.
E-mail address: dmeaney@emory.edu

Obstet Gynecol Clin N Am 40 (2013) 475–512
http://dx.doi.org/10.1016/j.ogc.2013.05.009
0889-8545/13/$ – see front matter Published by Elsevier Inc.

Table 1
Classifications of genetic risk for breast cancer[a]

Sporadic	Familial	Hereditary
Single occurrence in family	Two or more first-degree or second-degree affected relatives	Multiple affected individuals in multiple generations
Late age of onset (after 60 y)	Onset typically after 50 y	Early age of onset (often less than 50 y)
Unilateral	Primarily unilateral or late-onset bilateral	Bilateral/multifocal disease
Lack of other cancers in the family, or only common cancers of late onset	Evidence of skipped generations, no clear inheritance pattern	Presence of ovarian cancer, male breast cancer, Jewish ancestry (suggests *BRCA1/2*); multiple other unusual and/or early onset malignancies
Primarily caused by age an other nongenetic factors	Multiple minor/moderate inherited genetic factors interacting with environment	Single major cancer susceptibility gene mutation, autosomal dominant inheritance

[a] Classifications are general and overlap can be seen, especially in small families with few female members (ie, limited family history).

approximately 2% to 7% of all breast cancers, and 10% to 15% of all ovarian cancers.[5–8] HBOC is associated with germline mutations in the *BRCA1* or *BRCA2* genes, isolated in 1994 and 1995 respectively.[9,10] Approximately 1 in 400 individuals in the general population, and 1 in 40 individuals of Ashkenazi Jewish descent, carry a mutation in one of these genes.[8,11–13]

Over the 2 decades since these genes were discovered and clinical testing has become available, a wealth of evidence has accumulated documenting the personal, familial, and population health advantages of identifying individuals at risk for HBOC, providing genetic counseling and testing, and offering enhanced surveillance and surgical risk reduction options. This article provides an overview of current knowledge and practice regarding HBOC. Practical information regarding collecting a family history, cancer genetic counseling, and testing is followed by a discussion of specific cancer risks in HBOC, cancer prognosis and treatment, screening recommendations, and risk reduction strategies. This resource for women's health providers, will assist in the identification of women and families affected by HBOC, and their clinical management.

THE IMPORTANCE OF FAMILY HISTORY

Despite the increasing availability of direct-to-consumer genetic testing and multigene panels, a detailed family history remains the most important and easily affordable tool for identifying individuals at familial or hereditary risk for breast, ovarian, or other cancers. Collecting a family history to identify possible HBOC should, at minimum, include the following:

- History of breast and/or ovarian cancer (cancer of the peritoneum and fallopian tubes should be considered a part of the spectrum of HBOC) in all:
  - First-degree relatives (parents, siblings, children), and
  - Second-degree relatives (aunts/uncles, grandparents, nieces/nephews)

- Both maternal and paternal sides of the family (Case Study 1)
- Age of diagnosis of the cancers, and
- Presence of Ashkenazi (eastern European) Jewish ancestry (Case Study 2)

Case Study 1. Importance of paternal family history

A 35-year-old woman presented to her physician with concerns about her risk for breast cancer. Her physician asked about history of breast cancer in her mother or sisters, and she reported none. The patient was diagnosed with stage II breast cancer 2 years later, at which time she was referred for genetic counseling and testing based on her young age. Her family history revealed that her father was diagnosed with prostate cancer at 58 years of age, a paternal aunt with breast cancer at 40 years of age, and a paternal first cousin with breast cancer at 45 years of age. Her paternal grandmother died at 55 years of age of so-called female cancer, which records later revealed was an ovarian primary. She ultimately tested positive for a *BRCA1* mutation.

Key points: *BRCA1/2* mutations are equally inherited through the paternal and maternal lineages. Focusing only on history of cancer in mothers and sisters, and not taking into account paternal family history and second-degree relatives, misses many patients at risk for HBOC.

Case Study 2. Epithelial ovarian cancer in an Ashkenazi Jewish family

A 30-year-old woman of Ashkenazi Jewish descent reported that her sister was recently diagnosed with stage IIIC epithelial ovarian cancer, serous type, at age 40 years. Her sister was advised to see a genetic counselor, but her condition deteriorated rapidly and she died before in-hospital genetic testing/DNA banking could be performed. The patient presented with concerns about her own risk of ovarian cancer and pursued genetic testing. She was found to carry a BRCA 1 mutation.

Key points: A single case of epithelial ovarian cancer can be a hallmark of HBOC, particularly in families of Ashkenazi Jewish descent. Genetic testing of an affected individual is the most informative. Given the prevalence of *BRCA* mutations in the Ashkenazi Jewish population and in serous ovarian cancer, genetic testing of an unaffected patient with a family history of epithelial ovarian cancer is indicated.

Cancer genetic professionals collect the following additional features in obtaining a comprehensive cancer pedigree for risk assessment, an example of which is shown in **Fig. 1**.

- Ancestry/ethnicity
- Both unaffected as well as affected individuals in the family and their ages/ages at death
- Bilateral or multifocal disease
- Cancer treatment (type of breast surgery, whether chemotherapy or hormone therapy given)
- Cancer pathology including hormone status
- History of previous preventive surgeries (oophorectomy, contralateral mastectomy)
- History of chemoprevention (oral contraceptives, tamoxifen)
- Other known HBOC-related cancers (eg, pancreatic, prostate, melanoma)
- Other cancers, benign tumors
- Relevant environmental exposures
- Prior genetic testing in the family

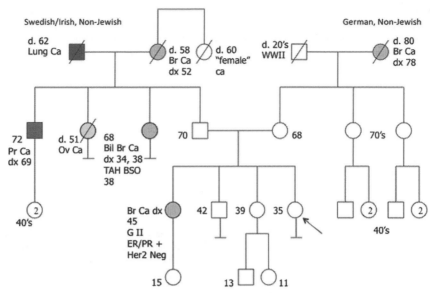

Fig. 1. Comprehensive cancer genetics pedigree. BSO, bilateral salpingo-oophorectomy; d., died; dx, diagnosed; ER/PR +, estrogen and progesterone receptor positive; G, grade; Pr, prostate; TAH, total abdominal hysterectomy.

Although collecting a complete cancer pedigree would be prohibitive in a primary care setting, red flags for HBOC that women's health practitioners should be aware of include:

- Early age of onset (50 years or younger for breast)
- Multiple affected first-degree or second-degree relatives (same side of family) in multiple generations with breast and/or ovarian cancer
- Bilateral breast cancer
- Breast and ovarian cancer in the same individual
- Male breast cancer
- Ashkenazi Jewish ancestry

Ovarian cancer is a stronger indication of HBOC than breast cancer, and, when referring to ovarian cancer in this article, fallopian tube and peritoneal cancers, which are considered part of the HBOC spectrum, are also included.[14–17] When *BRCA1* and *BRCA2* were first identified, it was thought that there also existed a separate gene or genes responsible for families with multiple cases of ovarian cancer, but no breast cancer. However, to date there has been no ovarian cancer–only gene identified, and most hereditary ovarian cancer families have been found to carry a *BRCA1* or *BRCA2* mutation. Because ovarian cancer is so much less common than breast cancer, the occurrence of 2 cases in the same family is significant, and even a single case may signal a *BRCA* mutation (see Case Study 2). Furthermore, although many breast cancers in HBOC occur before the age 50 years, most ovarian cancer associated with *BRCA1/2* mutations occurs between the ages of 50 and 70 years.[18] Thus, a woman whose mother and maternal grandmother had ovarian cancer at ages 55 and 60 years, respectively, has a greater risk for breast cancer than a woman whose mother and maternal grandmother were diagnosed with breast cancer in their 40s, because she is at higher risk to carry a *BRCA* mutation (18% vs 5% using the

BRCAPRO model, described later). The single strongest predictor of a *BRCA1/2* mutation is the presence of both a primary breast cancer and a primary ovarian cancer in the same individual.

GUIDELINES

Several organizations have developed guidelines or recommendations regarding HBOC identification, testing, and management. In 2005 the United States Preventive Services Task Force (USPSTF) released a grade B recommendation indicating that "women whose family history is associated with an increased risk for deleterious mutations in *BRCA1* or *BRCA2* genes be referred for genetic counseling and evaluation for *BRCA* testing."[19] The USPSTF outlined specific family history patterns associated with an increased risk for deleterious *BRCA* mutations, and estimated that 2% of adult women in the general population would have an increased-risk family history according to their definition.[19] The USPSTF is currently updating and revising these recommendations, which are anticipated to be released in the spring of 2013.

In 2009, the American College of Obstetrics and Gynecology (ACOG) released a practice bulletin regarding HBOC.[20] The bulletin provided 2 sets of criteria, one indicating patients with a greater than an approximate 20% to 25% chance of having a *BRCA1/2* mutation in whom genetic risk assessment is recommended, and a second indicating patients with greater than an approximate 5% to 10% chance of having a *BRCA1/2* mutation in whom genetic risk assessment may be helpful.[20] Although these recommendations align with those of the Society of Gynecologic Oncologists published in 2007,[21] restricting genetic risk assessment to women with a 20% or greater likelihood would miss a substantial number of individuals who are at risk for HBOC. As evidence has accumulated regarding the benefit of identification and management of individuals with HBOC, there has been trend toward offering genetic testing to women with lower mutation probabilities.

The National Comprehensive Cancer Network (NCCN) recommendations on "Genetic/Familial High Risk Assessment: Breast and Ovarian" (http://www.nccn.org/professionals/physician_gls/pdf/genetics_screening.pdf) are widely used and include criteria for genetic risk evaluation, as well as HBOC testing criteria and management recommendations. The NCCN recommendations are the most updated and comprehensive, and most likely to be followed by cancer genetics professionals. Of the three sets of guidelines mentioned thus far, NCCN is most likely to capture the highest percentage of individuals with a *BRCA* mutation. For example, any history of breast cancer before the age of 45 years (or breast cancer at age 50 years or younger if limited family history); triple-negative breast cancer at age 60 years or younger; male breast cancer; or epithelial ovarian cancer in the patient, first-degree relative, or second-degree relative are considered criteria for genetic testing.[22]

Although there is overlap among these guidelines, none of the criteria provided have been prospectively evaluated with respect to positive or negative predictive values. The NCCN criteria likely have high sensitivity, but specificity may be low, because the likelihood of a *BRCA* mutation is present in non-Jewish unaffected individuals with a single first-degree or second-degree relative with early onset breast cancer or ovarian cancer is less than 3% (as modeled using BRCAPRO). Although such unaffected individuals may be appropriate candidates for referral, providers should be cautious about ordering direct testing without first referring the patient for comprehensive cancer risk assessment by a qualified individual. In all cases, *BRCA* testing is most useful, informative, and appropriate if performed first on an individual with a personal history of breast and/or ovarian cancer.

The complexity of the ACOG and NCCN criteria may pose a challenge for a busy practitioner trying to determine which patients to refer to cancer genetic professionals for risk assessment and counseling regarding *BRCA* testing. A few online referral screening tools have been developed to facilitate this process. Both the Pedigree Assessment Tool (PAT; https://myosfhealth.osfhealthcare.org/sites/OSF/BCRA/Web_Pages/bcra.aspx) and the Breast Cancer Genetics Referral Screening Tool (B-RST; www.breastcancergenescreen.org) have been clinically validated against more complex risk models requiring detailed pedigrees and computer entry.[23–26] Although Myriad Genetic Laboratories, Inc, have a hereditary cancer quiz on their Web site (www.hereditarycancerquiz.com/), no validation data are available and, given that it is nonspecific, the use of this quiz would likely result in significant over-referral or testing of low-risk women. As with any screening modality, the effectiveness of these tools lies in an appropriate balance between sensitivity and specificity, while maintaining ease of use.

Practitioners should be aware that the frequently used Gail model[27] fails to detect a substantial number of women at risk for HBOC, because it only considers breast cancer in mothers and sisters, does not adjust for age of onset or bilaterality, and does not take into consideration ovarian cancer in the family.[26] As such, it should not be used to determine who should be referred for genetic counseling or *BRCA* testing.

CANCER GENETIC RISK ASSESSMENT AND COUNSELING

The importance of appropriate cancer genetic risk assessment, as well as pretest and posttest counseling provided by appropriately trained individuals, has been emphasized by multiple organizations including the USPSTF, the NCCN, and the Commission on Cancer in their 2012 guidelines.[19,22,28] Comprehensive cancer risk assessment includes the completion of a detailed cancer pedigree, and use of appropriate validated models to assess the likelihood of an individual carrying a *BRCA1/2* mutation, as well as the individual's personal cancer risks. Of particular importance, cancer risk assessment performed by a genetic counselor or other similarly trained health care provider may be able to determine who in the family the most appropriate person to test to maximize the information obtained. Furthermore, comprehensive cancer risk assessment can identify a patient's risk for other cancers, or may identify that a different hereditary cancer syndrome should be considered in the differential diagnosis. **Box 1** lists the key components in the provision of comprehensive cancer genetics risk assessment, counseling, and testing, based on guidelines and recommendations from ACOG, the American Society of Clinical Oncology, and the National Society of Genetic Counselors.[20,29–31]

Several models have been developed and validated to assist in assessing an individual's likelihood to carry a *BRCA1/2* mutation and their associated risk for breast and/or ovarian cancer. The most commonly used models are presented in **Table 2**. No single model is ideal, and the results they provide are only as good as the completeness and accuracy of the input information. They should not be relied on exclusively to determine who should or should not be offered genetic testing. An appropriately trained genetic health care provider also uses additional information contained in a complete pedigree, such as size of the family, number of female relatives, presence of cancers not included in the model (eg, pancreatic, prostate, melanoma), missing information, and details regarding pathology, previous preventive

| Box 1 |
| Steps involved in risk assessment, genetic counseling, and testing for HBOC |

1. Collect and document patient and family cancer and relevant health history
2. Analyze/interpret patient and family health histories to determine:
   - Likelihood of a *BRCA1/2* mutation (for patient, in family)
   - Possibility of a different hereditary cancer syndrome
   - Mutation-based and empirical cancer risks
3. Assess psychosocial and interpersonal dynamics
4. Educate patient regarding:
   - Basic principles of cancer genetics
   - Cancer risks associated with *BRCA1/2* mutations
   - Autosomal dominant inheritance of *BRCA1/2* mutations
   - Personal mutation probability and cancer risks
5. Facilitate informed consent through discussion of the availability, limitations, risk, and benefits of *BRCA1/2* testing, including:
   - Most appropriate testing strategy
   - Possible test results and their implications
   - Genetic discrimination, confidentiality, and protective laws
   - Screening and risk reduction strategies and their effectiveness
   - Psychosocial impact on self/family members
   - Cost/insurance coverage
6. Disclose, interpret, and discuss test results
   - Impact of result on personal cancer risks
   - Medical management recommendations
   - Implications for family members
   - Psychosocial response
7. Follow-up
   - Support resources
   - Referrals for medical management
   - Opportunities for research participation
   - Documentation for family members and care providers

surgeries, and so forth, to assist in the risk assessment process. The wide variation in *BRCA* mutation probability calculated by these models is shown in **Fig. 2.**

GENETIC TESTING FOR HBOC

At present, there is only 1 company in the United States that offers complete testing for mutations in the *BRCA1/2* genes: Myriad Genetic Laboratories, Inc, which holds a controversial patent on performing *BRCA1/2* molecular analysis.[32] The type of testing offered, and the completeness of the testing, has changed significantly over the past

Table 2
HBOC risk calculation models

Model	Parameters Considered	Output	Comments
BOADICEA https://pluto.srl.cam.ac.uk/cgi-bin/bd2/v2/bd.cgi	History of breast and ovarian cancer in first-degree, second-degree, and third-degree relatives; male breast cancer; age at diagnosis; bilateral breast cancer; breast and ovarian cancer in same person; unaffected relatives; AJ ancestry; pancreatic and prostate cancer	Probability of a *BRCA1/2* mutation; breast and ovarian cancer age-adjusted cumulative risks	Detailed pedigree information required; data entry time consuming and complex; allows for non-*BRCA1/2* genetic effects
BRCAPRO http://www4.utsouthwestern.edu/breasthealth/cagene/	History of breast and ovarian cancer in first-degree and second-degree relatives; male breast cancer; age at diagnosis; bilateral breast cancer; breast and ovarian cancer in same person; unaffected relatives; AJ ancestry; breast cancer pathology results; prior oophorectomy	Probability of a *BRCA1/2* mutation; breast and ovarian cancer age-adjusted cumulative risks based on mutation probability; also provides Claus, Gail, and other hereditary cancer models	Detailed pedigree information required; adjusts for unaffected family members; uses high penetrance estimates; does not incorporate third-degree relatives and half-siblings
IBIS http://www.ems-trials.org/riskevaluator/	Breast cancer and age at onset in first-degree, second-degree, and third-degree relatives; ovarian cancer and age at onset in first-degree and second-degree relatives; bilateral breast cancer in first-degree relatives; Jewish ancestry Nongenetic factors: age at menarche, parity, age at first live birth, age at menopause, use of hormone replacement therapy, benign breast disease (hyperplasia, atypical hyperplasia, LCIS), height (premenopausal), BMI (postmenopausal)	Probability of a *BRCA1/2* mutation; age-adjusted cumulative breast cancer risk compared with population in graph form	Incorporates both genetic and nongenetic risk factors Easy data entry, but requires extensive family history details

Model	Input	Output	Limitations
Myriad II http://www.myriadtests.com/provider/brca-mutation-prevalence.htm (also available within BRCAPRO)	History of breast and ovarian cancer in first-degree and second-degree relatives; age of diagnosis in broad categories; male breast cancer; AJ ancestry	Probability of a *BRCA1/2* mutation	Limited number of affected family members included; age of diagnosis only in broad categories; unaffected not accounted for; family history data obtained from test requisition forms and thus possibly limited/biased
Penn II http://www.afcri.upenn.edu/itacc/penn2/	Numbers of: breast cancers before age 50 y, ovarian cancers, bilateral breast cancers, individuals with both breast and ovarian cancer, male breast cancer, prostate cancer, youngest age of breast cancer diagnosis, presence of pancreatic cancer in family, AJ ancestry, closest affected relative	Probability of a *BRCA1/2* mutation for patient and family	Easy entry; does not incorporate all family history information (eg, breast cancers at ≥50 y), specific ages of diagnosis, unaffected individuals

First-degree relatives are parents, siblings, and children; second-degree relatives are grandparents, aunts/uncles, and nieces/nephews; third-degree relatives are cousins and great grandparents.

Abbreviations: AJ, Ashkenazi Jewish; BMI, body mass index; LCIS, lobular carcinoma in situ.

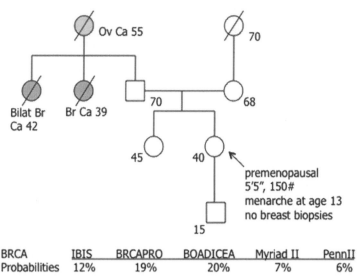

BRCA	IBIS	BRCAPRO	BOADICEA	Myriad II	PennII
Probabilities	12%	19%	20%	7%	6%

Fig. 2. Comparison of BRCA probability models. Bilat, bilateral; Br, breast; Ca, cancer; Ov, ovarian.

decade. **Table 3** lists the currently available testing options, how they differ, and, most importantly, indications for use and limitations.

Possible Test Results and Interpretation

Test result interpretation depends not only on the result itself but also on which person in the family was tested, whether the person tested was affected with breast or ovarian cancer, and the type of test ordered. As mentioned previously, testing is most informative for the patient and the family if first performed on someone with a personal history of breast and/or ovarian cancer. When considering the family in **Fig. 1**, the most appropriate individual to test first is the maternal aunt with early onset bilateral breast cancer, because she has the highest probability to carry a mutation.

Positive

A positive result is indicated by the identification of a known deleterious mutation in *BRCA1* or *BRCA2* (ie, one that disrupts normal protein function and is associated with increased risks for breast, ovarian, and other related cancers). Analytical validity is high and thus false-positives are not expected with *BRCA* testing given the methodology used. Based on autosomal dominant inheritance (see Case Study 1), all first-degree relatives have an a priori 50% likelihood to also carry the same mutation.

True negative

Once a mutation has been identified in a family, it allows highly accurate testing of other biological family members. Any family member of an identified mutation carrier, who subsequently is found not to carry this same mutation on single-site analysis, is considered a true-negative. This individual is unlikely to be at increased risk for breast/ovarian or related cancers beyond that of the general population (assuming no personal nongenetic risk factors, or significant cancer history on the other side of the family).[33–35] In a sense, it is as if this person's strong family history no longer influences the risk. As such, women receiving a true-negative result are recommended to undergo

Table 3
BRCA1/2 available testing

Test Name	What It Does	Indications for Use	Comments
Integrated BRACAnalysis[a]	Full sequencing and deletion/duplication (large rearrangement) analysis of both BRCA1 and BRCA2	Non-Jewish, first person in the family to be tested, ideally someone with a history of breast or ovarian cancer	Most comprehensive and most expensive. Still misses rare/currently unidentifiable mutations. New, so may not be covered by all insurance carriers who cover testing
Comprehensive BRACAnalysis	Full sequencing of BRCA1 and BRCA2, evaluation for 5 common deletions/duplications in BRCA1 (5-site rearrangement panel)	First person in the family to be tested: ideally someone with a history of breast or ovarian cancer	Detects 92.5%[b] mutations in BRCA1/2. Misses large rearrangements other than the 5 evaluated
Multisite 3 BRACAnalysis	Tests only for presence/absence of the 3 Ashkenazi Jewish founder mutations: BRCA1: 5385insC, 187delAG BRCA2: 6174delT	Appropriate first test for individual of Ashkenazi Jewish descent with a personal history of breast or ovarian cancer, or history of breast/ovarian cancer on the side of the family with Jewish ancestry. Even if a founder mutation has been identified in a family, the Multisite 3 should be ordered on other family members, particularly if both sides are of Ashkenazi Jewish descent	Detects about 95% of mutations in individuals of Ashkenazi Jewish ancestry. If there is a strong personal or family history, should consider reflexing to comprehensive/integrated analysis
Single-site BRACAnalysis	Tests for presence or absence of a single specified mutation in BRCA1 or BRCA2	Used when a biological family member has previously been found to carry this mutation	Highly accurate and informative within a family
BART	Tests for large rearrangements in BRCA1/BRCA2 which are not identified by Comprehensive BRACAnalysis	May be appropriate reflex test if no mutation identified by Comprehensive BRACAnalysis	Yield is low if there is not a strong family history.[c] May not be covered as additional test by some insurers

Abbreviation: BART, BRACAnalysis rearrangement test.

[a] Testing recently changed from comprehensive to integrated (early 2013) in response to a change in NCCN guidelines released in 2012 recommending that all patients undergo the large rearrangement panel (BART).

[b] Eighty percent among individuals of Latin American/Caribbean ancestry.

[c] Exception for individuals of Latin American/Caribbean ancestry, in whom 20% of mutations are identified by BART. Evidence suggests a higher prevalence of large rearrangements in patients of Near/Middle Eastern descent as well.

general population screening.[33] Furthermore, their children have no chance of maternally inheriting the mutation, and therefore do not have increased risks for BRCA-related cancers. However, it is important for these individuals to understand that this does not eliminate the chance that they could develop breast or ovarian cancer, because they are still subject to the background general population risk.

Uninformative negative

If no prior mutation has been identified in a family, negative BRCA testing on an individual is considered to be an uninformative negative. Interpretation of such a result again depends on who was tested, and which test was performed. If an individual without a personal history of breast/ovarian cancer tests negative, this could be explained by several factors: (1) there is a BRCA mutation in the family that the person tested did not inherit, (2) this is not an HBOC family, (3) the patient carries a BRCA mutation that was not identified by the test performed, (4) there is a mutation in a different hereditary cancer gene, and (5) the cancer in the family is the result of minor genetic susceptibility factors (familial cancer). In this last circumstance, the patient's risk for cancer is reduced, but remains increased beyond that of the general population. If an individual with a personal history of breast or ovarian cancer tests negative, residual risks for this to be an HBOC family are lower, but again not eliminated depending on which test was performed. In some situations, the person with cancer who was tested represents a phenocopy (ie, they had breast cancer because of chance or other factors, and there may still be a mutation in the family), which emphasizes why it is important to first test the individual with the highest a priori likelihood to carry a mutation. For families whose history strongly suggests HBOC, it may be appropriate to pursue testing on a second affected individual. Furthermore, when working with individuals who underwent BRCA testing in the past with an uninformative negative result, the practitioner should determine whether or not large rearrangement testing (BRACAnalysis rearrangement test [BART]) was performed. In some cases, it may be appropriate to offer this as additional testing. Revaluation and consideration of further testing should also occur if additional family members are diagnosed with relevant cancers.

Variant of uncertain significance

The most challenging result to interpret is when a variant of uncertain significance (VUS) is identified. VUS means that a change in the DNA sequence of BRCA1 or BRCA2 was found, but it is unknown whether it affects protein function (ie, whether it is deleterious). Such findings are common, occurring in 5% to 10% of test cases in general, although in higher frequencies among certain ethnic groups such as African Americans (see Case Study 3).[5] In most cases, such variants are later classified as benign and, as such, a VUS result should not be interpreted as conferring an increased risk for breast/ovarian cancer. In some cases, the variant is further classified as favor polymorphism, indicating that evidence points to it being a benign change, or it may be classified as suspected deleterious. In the latter circumstance, there is substantial evidence to suggest that the variant disrupts normal protein function, but one or more lines of evidence is lacking to make this determination with certainty. Clinicians should interpret and act on VUS results cautiously, taking into account personal history, family history, and available information about the variant. Preventive surgery for an individual prompted by a VUS finding alone is not recommended, unless the variant is classified as suspected deleterious, and then only after careful counseling. Although most suspected deleterious variants are later reclassified as true disease-causing mutations, there have been a few cases in which they were downgraded to benign polymorphisms. Myriad Genetic Laboratories, Inc, carefully monitors information regarding VUSs and, in circumstances in which a variant is reclassified, addended reports are sent to the ordering clinician of any patient who previously was found to carry the variant. Given the frequency with which patients change health care providers, clinicians need to emphasize to patients receiving a VUS result the importance of periodic genetic reassessment to update information regarding their genetic status.

Case Study 3. VUSs

A 29-year-old African American woman presents for a routine examination with a new provider. Because her mother's death was caused by breast cancer at 45 years of age, the patient's doctor ordered *BRCA* testing. The patient was found to carry a VUS in the *BRCA2* gene and the results were relayed to her over the telephone. She consulted a surgeon, whom she told about her mother's history and her positive *BRCA* test results and requested a prophylactic mastectomy (PM). A year after her surgery, she received a letter in the mail telling her that the variant had been reclassified to a benign polymorphism.

Key points: VUSs are common, especially among African Americans, in whom they are found in 15% to 20% of individuals tested. Careful pretest counseling about the possibility of a VUS, and appropriate posttest counseling and investigation regarding possible significance of the VUS, are critical to preventing anxiety and unnecessary medical interventions.

Other Genetic Risk Factors for Breast Cancer

Although *BRCA1/2* mutations account for most hereditary breast cancers, less common mutations in other high-penetrance genes also predispose to breast and other cancers (**Table 4**).[36,37] In addition, genetic testing is now available for some moderate-penetrance genes such as *CHEK2, ATM, NBS1, RAD50, BRIP1,* and *PALB2.*[36–38] Mutations in these genes are associated with a 2-fold to 4-fold increased risk for breast cancer, and are estimated to account for 2% to 4% of familial breast cancer.[36–38] However, the clinical usefulness of testing for mutations in these genes remains unclear, because data regarding the implications of finding a mutation in an individual are limited with respect to impact on medical management or impact of a negative result on cancer risks in family members.[36]

Some testing companies have recently begun to offer panels that use next-generation sequencing to screen for mutations in multiple genes, both of high and moderate penetrance (eg, www.ambrygen.com/tests/breastnext). However, such

---

Table 4
Other hereditary cancer syndromes predisposing to breast cancer[a]

Condition	Gene(s)	Breast Cancer Risks	Other Associated Cancers
Li-Fraumeni syndrome	*TP53*	56% by age 45, >90% lifetime	Soft tissue sarcomas, leukemias, brain tumors, osteosarcomas, adrenal cancers
Cowden syndrome	*PTEN*	30%–50% lifetime	Thyroid, endometrial cancers
Peutz-Jeghers syndrome	*STK11*	8% by age 40 y, 32% by age 60 y	Colorectal, gastric, pancreatic cancers
Hereditary diffuse gastric cancer	*CDH1*	(Lobular) 39% lifetime	Diffuse gastric cancer

[a] These syndromes account for less than 1% of breast cancers.[201]

panels cannot, at this point, include *BRCA1/2* testing because of the Myriad patent. Furthermore, in addition to the uncertain clinical usefulness of testing for moderate-penetrance genes, there is a substantial likelihood that a VUS will be found in one or more of the genes tested. Although pursuing a multigene panel in an individual with a suggestive personal/family history who is negative for a *BRCA1/2* mutation is a consideration, it must be accompanied by careful counseling regarding the probability of a VUS and the unknown management implications of finding a mutation in some of the genes included. Consultation with a cancer genetics professional is encouraged for any patient for whom a multigene panel is being considered.

In addition, clinicians should be aware of the genetic testing for breast cancer risk currently being offered direct to consumers (DTC) by such companies as 23andMe. These breast cancer genomic risk profiles look for single nucleotide polymorphisms (SNPs) that have been found in genome-wide association studies to be associated with breast cancer. However, the relative risk associated with these SNPs is low (1.1-fold to 1.4-fold), the risk predictions may not incorporate family history or other risk factors, and thus their predictive ability is limited.[39,40] Furthermore, 23andMe reports on 3 SNPs linked to the *BRCA1/2* Ashkenazi Jewish founder mutations, which may lead to both uncertainty and anxiety if consumers learn that they carry *BRCA* mutations without having had the benefit of pretest counseling. Individuals undergoing DTC testing may also be falsely reassured that they are not at risk for HBOC because they tested negative for the BRCA-associated SNPs, or were low risk on the panel.

CHALLENGES AND BARRIERS ASSOCIATED WITH GENETIC COUNSELING AND TESTING FOR HBOC

Multiple factors have been shown to pose challenges to both referral and use of cancer risk counseling and testing for *BRCA1/2* mutations. These factors include cost and insurance coverage, provider awareness, race/ethnicity, concerns regarding insurance discrimination, and psychosocial barriers.[37,41–44] Although affordability of *BRCA* testing and insurance coverage remain a barrier for some women,[43] many private insurance companies now cover genetic counseling and testing for *BRCA1/2* mutations. However, which level of testing is covered, and what patient/family history characteristics qualify a patient for coverage, varies by provider and plan. Starting in 2014, provisions of the Affordable Care Act will require Medicare and all qualified commercial health insurers (except grandfathered individual and employer-sponsored plans) to pay for genetic counseling and *BRCA* testing as preventive care, given that these services have received a grade B recommendation from the USPSTF.[45] Medicare currently pays for genetic testing in patients with a personal history of breast or ovarian cancer meeting specified criteria. Coverage by Medicaid is inconsistent, with some state programs covering testing and others not. Myriad offers a financial hardship program to assist patients without insurance coverage in obtaining *BRCA* testing; however, this program is not available to Medicaid recipients or patients who have other insurance, even if genetic testing is not covered.

In addition to issues of cost, concerns regarding potential insurance discrimination inhibit some patients from seeking cancer genetic counseling and testing services, and also inhibit some providers from referring patients for such services.[44] Despite the fear, there are few documented cases of patients either losing health insurance or being denied coverage because of a genetic test result.[46] Most states currently have laws in place that prohibit health insurers from denying coverage or charging higher rates based on genetic test results or information. In addition, the

Genetic Information Non-Discrimination Act (GINA), passed in 2009, prohibits both health insurance and employment discrimination resulting from genetic information.[46] The Affordable Care Act will provide further protection beginning in 2014 because insurers will not be able to use preexisting conditions in coverage or rate decisions.[47] However, currently there is no legal protection from genetic discrimination by life or long-term/disability insurance companies. In this regard, an important part of the pretest counseling process is to encourage the patient to consider whether they wish to purchase life or disability insurance for themselves or their children before testing.

The psychosocial impact of hereditary cancer genetic testing has been well studied. Contrary to concerns raised when *BRCA* testing first became available in 1996, there is little evidence to suggest that undergoing genetic counseling and testing for *BRCA* mutations, or receipt of a positive genetic test result, leads to substantial increases in depression or anxiety.[48] It has been shown that, in families with known *BRCA* mutations, it is those individuals who choose not to undergo testing who have the greatest levels of anxiety and depression.[49] In addition, many women who undergo *BRCA* testing are from families in which they have witnessed the impact of breast or ovarian cancer on multiple female relatives. These women are often empowered by knowing their mutation status and being able to pursue screening and preventive measures that have been shown to be lifesaving (although there may be still emotional implications when a *BRCA* mutation is identified within a family). Mutation carrier parents may experience feelings of guilt at having passed the mutation to their children, and family members found not to carry the mutation may experience survival guilt in relation to their relatives who tested positive.[50] These issues point to the importance of adequately addressing psychosocial and family issues in the pretest and posttest counseling sessions.[29,35,48] **Box 2** provides links to support resources for individuals and families affected by HBOC, as well as Web sites for locating cancer genetics professionals.

Box 2
Resources

To locate a cancer genetics professional:

- National Society of Genetic Counselors. http://www.nsgc.org/FindaGeneticCounselor/tabid/64/Default.aspx

- National Cancer Institute Cancer Genetics Services Directory. http://www.cancer.gov/search/geneticsservices/

- National Institutes of Health Gene Tests. http://www.ncbi.nlm.nih.gov/sites/GeneTests/clinic

Patient resources:

- Facing our Risk for Cancer Empowered (FORCE); an excellent resource for individuals at potential hereditary risk for breast/ovarian cancer: http://facingourrisk.org

- Be Bright Pink; a resource for young women at high risk for breast/ovarian cancer: http://www.BeBrightPink.org/

- Young Survival Coalition; a resource for young women diagnosed with breast cancer: http://www.youngsurvival.org/

- Sharsheret; for young women and their families of all Jewish backgrounds facing breast cancer: http://www.sharsheret.org/

BREAST CANCER IN HBOC

A key feature of HBOC-associated breast cancer is that it often occurs in young women.[22] Although the average age of onset varies, HBOC should be considered in any woman who develops breast cancer before the age of 45 years.[22] Although large prospective studies are needed, some data also suggest that, as *BRCA* genetic mutations are passed down within a family, individuals of later generations may develop breast cancer at earlier ages.[51] Young age of onset may factor into decision making about the timing of preventive strategies among carriers. However, variation exists within families and therefore cumulative risks of breast cancer based on current age may provide important information to guide these decisions.

Women with *BRCA1/2* mutations have a substantially higher lifetime risk for breast cancer compared with women in the general population. Early risk estimates for *BRCA* mutation carriers, based on data from highly penetrant families, were as high as 84% by age 70 years.[52,53] More recent data derived from larger population-based studies suggest lower risks (45%–65%) by age 70 years.[54] **Fig. 3** shows the estimated cumulative risks of breast and ovarian cancer in *BRCA1* and *BRCA2* mutation carriers by age. Although these data are important, short-term age-adjusted risk for women presenting at different ages may be more informative in developing an individualized management plan. **Table 5** shows *BRCA1* and *BRCA2* breast cancer risks for 2 women of different ages, one at age 20 years and another at age 40 years; higher 10-year, 20-year, and 30-year risks are shown in the older woman. However, the older woman has a lower lifetime risk, because the longer a woman survives cancer free, the less likely she is to develop cancer. Women's health providers who understand these age-adjusted risks can assist women as they choose between enhanced surveillance, chemoprevention, and risk-reducing surgery throughout their lifespans.[55,56] Age-related risks are particularly relevant for young carriers, who may overestimate their short-term risk and consider aggressive surgery at young ages, even if it means they will forgo childbearing.[57] To assist carriers and their providers in understanding cancer risks by age, a simulation model is now available as an online tool (http://brcatool.stanford.edu). This software provides an interactive platform that evaluates

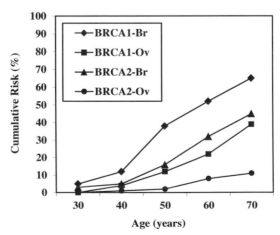

Fig. 3. Cumulative risks of breast and ovarian in BRCA 1/2 mutation carriers. (*Data from* Antoniou A, Pharoah PD, Narod S, et al. Average risks of breast and ovarian cancer associated with BRCA1 or BRCA2 mutations detected in case Series unselected for family history: a combined analysis of 22 studies. Am J Hum Genet 2003;72(5):1117–30.)

Table 5
Breast cancer risks by age

Risk to Develop Breast Cancer	Women Aged 20 y			Women Aged 40 y		
	BRCA1 (%)	BRCA2 (%)	Population Risk (%)	BRCA1 (%)	BRCA2 (%)	Population Risk (%)
10 y	1–2	1–1.5	0.1	16–25	12–19	1.5
20 y	10–14	6–10	0.5	31–45	24–36	4.1
30 y	24–35	17–26	1.9	41–58	34–49	7.6

Data from Chen S, Parmigiani G. Meta-analysis of BRCA1 and BRCA2 penetrance. J Clin Oncol 2007;25(11):1329–33; and National Cancer Institute, Surveillance Research, Cancer Control and Population Science. DevCan-Probability of Developing of Dying of Cancer. Available at: http://surveillance.cancer.gov/devcan/. Accessed March 1, 2013.

risk by age and calculates the risk reductions afforded by various clinical management decisions.[58,59]

BRCA mutation carriers who have developed breast cancer continue to face a higher risk for a second primary breast cancer, either ipsilateral or contralateral, than noncarriers. In early studies, the cumulative risk of a second breast cancer was estimated at 65% by age 70 years.[52] More recent data suggest that the risk is lower, approximately 40% (95% confidence interval [CI], 34.1%–47%) lifetime risk by age 70 years,[60] with a 12% to 27% risk within 5 years of the initial breast cancer diagnosis.[61] These risks may be higher for *BRCA1* carriers compared with *BRCA2* carriers.[61,62] Risk estimates for a second breast cancer (ipsilateral or contralateral) affect decisions about surgical options as treatment of breast cancer, as well as for prophylaxis. Recent trends suggest that many women are choosing contralateral mastectomy at the time of initial breast cancer diagnosis.[63]

Several factors may influence the risk of a second breast cancer among carriers. Older age at initial breast cancer diagnosis confers a lower risk of a second cancer, particularly when comparing those diagnosed before age 40 years with those diagnosed after age 50 years.[64] The use of adjuvant tamoxifen[65] and chemotherapy[66] have also been reported to reduce the risk of second breast cancers in carriers. This observed decrease is likely related to chemotherapy-induced early menopause and the reduction in hormonal influences afforded by menopause and tamoxifen use. Induction of menopause is also thought to be responsible for the lower rates of second cancers seen among carriers who have undergone oophorectomy.[61]

Male Breast Cancer

Although it is beyond the scope of this article to discuss the clinical management of male breast cancer, it is important emphasize the importance of genetic counseling and testing for male relatives. Because male breast cancer is so uncommon, it is considered a red flag for HBOC, and a single case in a family is considered a reason for genetic referral, regardless of age at diagnosis. Male breast cancer is most likely to be associated with a mutation in *BRCA2* and estimates indicate that male carriers have a 2.8% risk of developing breast cancer by age 70 years (95% CI, 0.6%–13%), which increases to 6.9% (95% CI, 1.2%–38.6%) by age 80 years.[67] This risk is substantially higher than the estimated population risk among noncarrier men, which has been reported as 1.08/100,000.[68] *BRCA1* mutations may also confer an increased risk for male breast cancer, although this is not universally accepted.[69]

Possible Mitigators of Breast Cancer Risk Among Carriers

Genetic factors

Most familial mutations in BRCA1/2 are unique, and genotype-phenotype correlations have not been delineated to the extent that they can be used reliably to alter clinical care. However, there is one region in BRCA2, known as the ovarian cancer cluster region, where mutations seem to confer a substantially higher risk of ovarian cancer than elsewhere in the gene.[67] To date, differentiating cancer risk based on location of mutations in the BRCA1 gene has been less conclusive.[60,69] Observed cancer rates differ between HBOC families, suggesting that other genetic modifiers, such as polymorphisms or mutations in other genes, may also influence cancer risk. One such modifier is a noncoding region of the RAD21 gene that has been shown to bind BRCA2 and is thought to increase the risk of breast cancer in BRCA carriers.[69–71]

Given that the specific genetic modifiers of risk are largely unknown, it has been suggested that family history may serve as a marker for specific risks within a family. Data from a prospective multinational cohort study suggest that risks are higher for mutation carriers with a first-degree relative with breast cancer less than 50 years old, or a first-degree or second-degree relative with ovarian cancer.[72] These findings suggest that either genetic modifiers and/or shared environmental/lifestyle factors are influencing risk.

Nongenetic factors

Reproductive and lifestyle factors are being investigated as potential modifiers of BRCA risk. Young age of menarche is a risk factor for sporadic breast cancer[73]; however, limited data exist in BRCA mutation carriers. One study showed that BRCA1 carriers who experienced menarche at age 14 to 15 years experienced a 54% lower risk of breast cancer risk compared with those with menarche at younger ages (≤11 years).[73]

There is conflicting data with respect to the effect of parity on breast cancer risk in BRCA mutation carriers. Some studies suggest an increased risk of early onset breast cancer with higher parity in BRCA1 and BRCA2 carriers.[74,75] However, a decrease in the risk of breast cancer in women of higher parity (>4 pregnancies) has also been observed in BRCA1 carriers compared with nulliparous women.[75] Age at first pregnancy may also confound the association between parity and breast cancer risk.[69]

Limited data suggest that breastfeeding for at least 1 year may reduce the risk of breast cancer among BRCA1 carriers. Longer breastfeeding intervals may increase the protective effect.[76] In contrast, the International BRCA1/2 Carrier Cohort Study did not show a risk reductive effect with breastfeeding in carriers.[77,78] Although there are a multitude of other benefits of breastfeeding for mother and infant that would not be expected to differ for mutation carriers, more data are needed to answer the question of impact on cancer risk.

Obesity and the amount of physical activity have also been suggested as possible mitigators of cancer risk in BRCA1/2 mutation carriers. Increased exercise levels and lack of obesity in adolescence were found to be associated with delayed breast cancer onset in women with BRCA mutations.[79] Also, weight loss early in life (ages 18–30 years) has been shown to reduce the risk of BRCA-associated breast cancer occurrence (odds ratio [OR], 0.47; 95% CI 0.28–0.79) between ages 30 and 49 years.[80]

Oral contraceptives

Breast cancer risk in BRCA carriers who use or have used oral contraceptives is limited by heterogeneous data and lack of consistent results. In a recent meta-analysis of oral contraceptive use in BRCA carriers, no significant increase in risk of breast cancer was observed in case-control data of *BRCA1/2* carriers.[81] However, in a subset of cohort studies identified in the review, an increased risk was observed among BRCA 1 carriers (OR, 1.48; 95% CI, 1.14–1.92),[81] a finding not seen when case-control or case-case studies were analyzed. A second meta-analysis reported no overall association of oral contraceptives and breast cancer risk (summary relative risk, 1.13; 95% CI, 0.88–1.45).[82] This study did report an increased risk with oral contraceptive formulations used before 1975, but no significant association could be found with current oral contraceptive formulations. Thus, although further studies involving *BRCA* mutation carriers are needed, the current data suggest the likelihood of a substantial increase in breast cancer with the use of current formulations of oral contraceptives is low. Studies have shown that ovarian cancer risk is decreased in oral contraceptive users (discussed later).

Prognosis in HBOC-associated Breast Cancer

Available studies indicate that breast cancers among women with *BRCA* mutations carries a similar prognosis to sporadic breast cancers, compared stage for stage, especially if chemotherapy is administered as part of the treatment.[83–85] However, BRCA mutation carriers have a higher risk for developing a second primary breast cancer.[86] Independent prognostic factors for survival in BRCA-associated breast cancer include tumor stage, adjuvant chemotherapy, histologic grade, estrogen-receptor status, and prophylactic oophorectomy.[85] However, prospective longitudinal studies are needed because most of the existing data are based on small numbers.[35] Although surgical decisions, such as mastectomy versus breast conservation, may be affected by identification of a *BRCA* mutation, carrier status does not at this time provide reliable prognostic or survival information.[35]

Pathologic Features

Breast cancer among *BRCA1* carriers tends to be mitotically active, of higher grade, and is commonly medullary type.[62,85] In addition, many breast tumors tend to lack estrogen and progesterone receptors and HER2/neu, and thus are labeled triple negative. In a recent study of BRCA 1 carriers, 78% were estrogen receptor negative, 79% were progesterone receptor negative, 90% were HER2/neu negative, and 69% were triple negative.[87] The pathologic characteristics of *BRCA2*-associated breast tumors are more heterogeneous. Overall they tend to be of higher grade, but have similar rates of estrogen receptor status compared with sporadic cancers.[88,89] *BRCA2*-associated breast cancer is more likely to lack overexpression of HER2/neu, although it is less likely to be triple negative.[87–89]

Treatment Differences

At present, the treatment options for breast cancer are not determined by *BRCA* status.[62] However, some studies have shown that women with breast cancer and a *BRCA* mutation are more likely to choose mastectomy, as well as prophylactic contralateral mastectomy, at the time of diagnosis.[90,91] Most studies do not show higher short-term local recurrence rates in carriers, although, as expected, long-term follow-up shows a higher likelihood of developing a second primary tumor, even within the treated breast.[92] Despite the increased risk of second primary breast cancer, available data have not indicated significant differences in overall survival.[85,93,94]

Some investigators suggest that *BRCA*-deficient breast cancers may respond differently to chemotherapy. The theory is that, because *BRCA* genes are involved in DNA repair, mutations in these genes may confer an increased sensitivity to chemotherapy. Small studies have found that *BRCA2* carriers, but not *BRCA1* carriers, have improved response rates to first-line chemotherapy (89% vs 50%; $P = .001$) including anthracyclines, cyclophosphamide, methotrexate, and fluorouracil. Better survival was demonstrated among BRCA2 carriers compared with noncarriers, but this was not observed in BRCA1 carriers.[95] A unique group of chemotherapeutic agents, poly (ADP-ribose) polymerase (PARP) inhibitors, are being evaluated to treat BRCA carriers, because they specifically target BRCA mutation pathways, preventing BRCA-mediated repair of DNA. Ongoing clinical trials using PARP inhibitors to treat breast cancer in BRCA mutation carriers have reported some preliminarily positive findings in patients with metastatic disease.[96]

Breast Cancer Screening

For women with HBOC, the approach to breast cancer screening and prevention differs from the general population. Because women with known BRCA mutations have a higher risk for breast cancer at younger ages (see **Table 5**), breast cancer screening is recommended earlier and is enhanced with the use of breast magnetic resonance imaging (MRI).[97] Annual mammograms alternating with MRI at 6-month intervals, beginning at age 25 years, are recommended (**Table 6**). Given the low sensitivity of mammography for young women with dense breasts[98] and concerns regarding cumulative radiation exposure beginning at age 25 years, the combined screening strategy of mammogram and MRI has recently been debated for women aged 25 to 30 years.[99] In clinical practice, some practitioners are delaying mammography screening until age 30 years, instead relying on screening with annual breast MRI for patients aged 25 to 30 years.[97,100,101] Alternating mammogram with MRI every 6 months beginning at age 30 years was recently shown to be cost-effective.[102] MRI has consistently been shown to have improved sensitivity compared with mammography in detecting breast cancer in carriers,[97,101,103–106] with a combined sensitivity of both tests of between 80% and 100%.[97] As with any screening methodology, MRI can result in false-positives; additional imaging, and possible surgical biopsy, may be required. Although lower than that of mammogram,[100] MRI has a high specificity rate,[97] approaching 95%, with an 11% rate of recall for additional imaging.[107] Studies report that women who have undergone combined MRI and mammogram screening had a rate of biopsy (percutaneous or surgical) between 5% and 11%.[97,104,107] These rates decrease with follow-up MRI screenings.[107]

For male BRCA carriers, breast cancer screening is recommended later than in women, with breast self-examination beginning at age 35 years. Clinical breast examination is also recommended beginning at this age, with a suggested frequency of every 6 to 12 months. Baseline mammogram can be considered in men at age 40 years and, depending on the baseline study, annual mammograms are recommended if gynecomastia or parenchymal/globular breast density is detected.[22]

Prophylactic Mastectomy

Multiple studies have shown substantial reduction in breast cancer incidence (>90%) in women with BRCA mutations undergoing PM.[108–111] Although the benefits of PM are widely accepted, the uptake of this preventive strategy among unaffected carriers varies; worldwide less then 20% of women choose this option.[112] However, for mutation carriers already diagnosed with unilateral breast cancer, many chose prophylactic contralateral mastectomy, typically with reconstruction, at the time of their initial diagnosis of breast cancer.[63]

Risk-reducing Salpino-oophorectomy

Risk-reducing salpingo-oophorectomy (RRSO) has been shown to reduce the risk of developing breast cancer in BRCA1/2 carriers by approximately 50%, with greater risk

Table 6
Clinical management of HBOC

Screening Test	Age (y)/Frequency	Comments
Breast awareness	Starting at age 18, periodic	Periodic, consistent self–breast examination may facilitate awareness and, for premenopausal women, may be most informative if performed at the completion of menses
CBE	Starting at age 25, every 6–12 mo	No controlled trials comparing CBE and no screening
Mammogram	Starting at age 25 or individualized based on earliest breast cancer in family, annually	Some data suggest that mammogram be added to MRI screening after age 30; additional studies are pending
Breast MRI	Starting at age 25 or individualized based on earliest breast cancer in family, annually	Preferable to perform on days 7–15 of cycle in premenopausal women
Chemoprevention: selective estrogen-receptor modulators	No age specified	Consider for breast cancer risk reduction; limited data exist on benefits in BRCA carriers (data are limited to tamoxifen only)
Risk-reducing mastectomy	No age specified	Counseling includes degree of protection, reconstruction, and risks
Chemoprevention: OC	No age specified	Consider for ovarian cancer risk reduction after discussion of risks and benefits; OCs acceptable for contraception
Bilateral RRSO	Recommended at age 35–40 and on completion of childbearing, or individualized based on earliest ovarian cancer in family	Counseling includes reproductive desires, cancer risks, degree of protection, menopausal symptoms, hormone replacement therapy, and related medical issues
CA-125/TVS	For patients who elect not to have RRSO starting at age 30 or 5–10 y before earliest ovarian cancer in family, every 6 mo	Data show that this screening strategy performed annually is not effective; limited data regarding the effectiveness of screening at 6-mo intervals. CA-125 preferably after day 5 of menstrual cycle in premenopausal women. TVS preferably days 1–10 of the cycle in premenopausal women

Abbreviations: CBE, clinical breast examination; OC, oral contraception; RRSO, risk-reducing salpingo-oophorectomy; TVS, transvaginal sonogram.

reduction for women who undergo the procedure before age 40 years.[111,113] In addition, there is an 80% to 95% reduction in ovarian cancer risk, as discussed later. Initial studies indicate a protective effect irrespective of whether the mutation is in *BRCA1* or *BRCA2*.[111,113] A recent study comparing the rates of breast cancer among *BRCA1/2* carriers suggest that, at least with short-term follow-up, a greater reduction in breast cancer risk is seen with RRSO among *BRCA2* carriers (72%) than among *BRCA1* carriers (39%).[114] However, a subsequent meta-analysis showed a similar risk reduction (approximate 50% reduction) for both *BRCA1* and *BRCA2* carriers.[115] Data have also shown improvements in breast cancer mortality with bilateral salpingo-oophorectomy.[108]

Chemoprevention

A large randomized trial showed that the use of tamoxifen for 5 years in women at increased risk for breast cancer was associated with a 50% reduction in breast cancer incidence compared with untreated controls.[116] In the subset of healthy *BRCA2* mutation carriers from this cohort, tamoxifen reduced the risk of breast cancer by 62%, although this effect was not seen for *BRCA1* carriers.[117] Tamoxifen has also been shown to decrease the risk for contralateral breast cancer in *BRCA* mutation carriers when given as adjuvant treatment.[118] The effect was equal in both *BRCA1* and *BRCA2* carriers, and seemed to prevent both ER-positive and ER-negative second breast cancers.[118] Few *BRCA* mutation carriers choose tamoxifen as the main risk reduction strategy because of fear of side effects.[112,119] The question of whether tamoxifen provides additional protection from a second primary breast cancer in patients who have undergone a prophylactic oophorectomy remains unresolved, with studies showing conflicting results.[61,118]

There are no available data evaluating the protective impact of raloxifene or aromatase inhibitors for the prevention of breast cancer among women who carry *BRCA* mutations. Some investigators speculate that these agents may be considered as additional chemoprevention for this population.[51,118] Studies of exemestane and letrozole as breast cancer prevention for BRCA mutation carriers are ongoing.[51] PARP inhibitors have also been proposed as possible chemoprevention.[120]

OVARIAN CANCER IN HBOC

Most HBOC families tend to have a preponderance of breast cancer compared with ovarian cancer, although exceptions do occur in families with mutations in the ovarian cancer cluster region of *BRCA2*.[69] However, a family history of ovarian cancer is one of the strongest risk factors for HBOC, with 8% to 13% of unselected ovarian cases showing *BRCA1* or *BRCA2* mutations.[121] Among ovarian cancer cases of the high-grade serous subtype, 16% to 21% of these women have *BRCA* mutations.[121] Women who carry a *BRCA* mutation are also at risk for fallopian tube and primary peritoneal cancer.[122,123]

BRCA1 and *BRCA2* mutations confer different risks of ovarian cancer and different ages of onset. The original Breast Cancer Linkage Consortium data indicated a 63% and 27% risk of ovarian cancer by age 70 years in *BRCA1* and *BRCA2* mutation carriers respectively,[53] whereas the risk for a mutation carrier with a previous diagnosis of breast cancer was estimated at 44% by age 70 years.[52] Newer risk estimates indicate that *BRCA1*-associated risks of ovarian cancer range from 39% to 46%, whereas *BRCA2*-associated risks are lower at 10% to 27%,[18,54,79,124] compared with the 1.8% risk of ovarian malignancy in the general population.[125]

The age of onset of ovarian cancer in women with *BRCA* mutations tends to be later than what is observed with breast cancer, particularly in *BRCA2* mutation carriers who are more likely to be diagnosed with ovarian cancer after age 50 years.[12,111] In addition, some studies suggest that *BRCA1* carriers are more likely to be diagnosed with ovarian cancer before age 50 years. **Table 7** shows the age-adjusted risks for ovarian cancer among *BRCA1* and *BRCA2* mutation carriers, in contrast with the risks in the general population.

Pathologic Features

BRCA-associated ovarian cancer is epithelial in origin and typically of high-grade serous pathology.[121] Mucinous, endometrioid, and clear cell types[126,127] have been shown in *BRCA* carriers; however, among studies of *BRCA*-associated cancers, serous adenocarcinomas were most common.[87,126] Like sporadic ovarian cancer, most *BRCA*-associated ovarian cancers are high grade, typically grade 3.[87] Pathologic evaluation of specimens obtained from patients who have undergone RRSO provide a window into the possible pathogenesis of BRCA-associated ovarian cancer. Early fallopian tube carcinomas and tubal intraepithelial carcinomas have been detected,[14,128,129] generating the hypothesis that the fimbria of the fallopian tubes may be the origin of BRCA-associated ovarian or peritoneal cancer.[14–16,35,129,130]

Prognosis

Epithelial ovarian cancers in *BRCA* mutation carriers are diagnosed at a younger age than sporadic ovarian cancers.[131] *BRCA1* mutations are more commonly seen in individuals with ovarian cancer diagnosed before the age of 50 years, and *BRCA2* mutations are often seen in women diagnosed with ovarian cancer before the age of 60 years.[12] However, patients with ovarian cancer with *BRCA* seem to have a better prognosis than patients with sporadic cancer.[132–135] Some studies suggest that patients with ovarian cancer with *BRCA2* mutations also have a better overall survival than *BRCA1* mutation carriers.[132,136,137] *BRCA*-associated ovarian, primary peritoneal, and fallopian tube cancer seem to be uniquely sensitive to chemotherapy, which may be responsible for the improved prognosis. Tumor biology may also play a role.[121,133] Differences in prognosis, as well as treatment, argue strongly that *BRCA* mutation testing should be performed routinely in all cases of high-grade ovarian cancer.[22]

Treatment

Studies of *BRCA*-associated epithelial ovarian, primary peritoneal, and fallopian tube cancer suggest that these tumors have an increased sensitivity to platinum-based

Table 7
Ovarian cancer risks by age

Risk to Develop Ovarian Cancer	Women Aged 20 y			Women Aged 40 y		
	BRCA1 (%)	BRCA2 (%)	Population Risk (%)	BRCA1 (%)	BRCA2 (%)	Population Risk (%)
10 y	1–2	<1	0	5–9	1–3	0.1
20 y	2–5	0.5–1.5	0.1	17–24	5–10	0.4
30 y	7–13	1–5	0.2	33–41	12–20	1.2

Data from Chen S, Parmigiani G. Meta-analysis of BRCA1 and BRCA2 penetrance. J Clin Oncol 2007;25(11):1329–33; and National Cancer Institute, Surveillance Research, Cancer Control and Population Science. DevCan-Probability of Developing of Dying of Cancer. Available at: http://surveillance.cancer.gov/devcan/. Accessed March 1, 2013.

chemotherapy.[121,133,138] PARP inhibitors have shown promise in the treatment of ovarian cancer and clinical trials are ongoing to assess potential benefits specifically in *BRCA* mutation carriers.[138–141] Based on findings thus far, many investigators have suggested that all patients with ovarian, primary peritoneal, and fallopian tube cancers should undergo *BRCA* testing to inform chemotherapeutic choices.[121,140,142]

Screening and Management

Unlike breast cancer, annual screening for ovarian cancer has not been shown to be effective in *BRCA* mutation carriers.[124,143,144] Screen-detected cancers are typically late stage, may represent incident or prevalent cases, and have developed between screenings. For women who have not completed childbearing, or who for other reasons elect not to undergo RRSO, concurrent screening with CA-125 and transvaginal sonogram every 6 months is an option beginning at age 30 years.[22] When there is a history of early onset ovarian cancer in the family, screening is recommended 5 to 10 years earlier than the youngest age of diagnoses (see **Table 6**).[22] Because screening at 6-month intervals has not proved effective, *BRCA* mutation carriers must be counseled regarding the limitations and should be educated about early symptoms of ovarian cancer to watch for during screening intervals.[22,145] Early ovarian cancers that have been detected with CA-125 and transvaginal ultrasound are typically those of low malignant potential or of nonepithelial origin, which are not considered part of the HBOC spectrum. It is currently unclear whether screening at semiannual intervals improves the sensitivity of these screening tests.[22]

Risk-Reducing Salpingo-oophorectomy

The mainstay for prevention of ovarian cancer in women with HBOC is RRSO, a procedure that has been shown in multiple studies to decrease the risk of ovarian, primary peritoneal, and fallopian tube cancer, with combined estimates indicating an 80% to 95% decrease in risk.[22,114,115,146] In addition to decreased incidence, reductions in breast cancer, ovarian cancer, and all-cause mortality associations with RRSO provide a further compelling argument for clinical benefit.[108] Hereditary ovarian cancers are rarely diagnosed before the age of 40 years,[131] thus the risk-benefit analysis weighs in favor of delaying RRSO until 35 to 40 years of age, once childbearing is complete. RRSO is widely accepted,[147] with low intraoperative and postoperative complication rates when performed laparoscopically.[148]

Occult malignancies have been discovered during RRSO, with an average prevalence of 4.4%.[128,146,149–152] Many of these cancers have been detected in the distal fallopian tube along with findings of tubal intraepithethial carcinoma on careful pathologic evaluation.[14,16,153,154] In addition, patients with fallopian tube cancers show a 16% to 30% prevalence of *BRCA* mutations.[14,16,130,153] Thus, serial sectioning of the fallopian tube and ovary should be performed at the time of RRSO, along with pelvic washings.[15,128,155,156] After RRSO, *BRCA* mutation carriers have a residual risk of primary peritoneal cancer, with cumulative risks estimated between 1% and 4.3% 20 years after the procedure.[146,150,157]

RRSO in premenopausal women results in an abrupt surgical menopause. Resulting menopausal symptoms can have an impact on health and quality of life[158–161] and should be discussed with *BRCA* mutation carriers before they choose to undergo the procedure. Women who undergo RRSO may also experience changes in sexual functioning[161] and may benefit from postoperative sexual counseling.[162] In addition, the influence of early hormone depletion on the risk of osteoporosis and heart disease is a concern.[160] Osteopenia and osteoporosis have been shown in BRCA mutation carriers after salpingo-oophorectomy, with higher rates detected in women who undergo the procedure before age 50 years.[160,163,164] However, thus far, increased fracture rates have not been shown[165,166] and age at menopause has little, if any, effect on hip fracture incidence.[167] Some studies have indicated an increased risk for cardiac disease and cardiac mortality in young women who experience surgical menopause.[168–170] However, in the large prospective cohort study, the Women's Health Initiative, women who underwent bilateral salpingo-oophorectomy before age 50 years did not show higher rates of heart disease or cardiovascular death than those who did not experience surgical menopause.[165] Most reassuring is that lower all-cause mortality has been observed in BRCA mutation carriers who have undergone RRSO compared with those who have not.[108]

Hysterectomy at the time of RRSO

Whether hysterectomy should be performed at the time of RRSO is controversial, suggesting the need for an individualized approach. A theoretic benefit of concurrent hysterectomy is the complete removal of the fallopian tube, including the interstitial portion, although to date malignancies arising from this section of the fallopian tube in *BRCA* carriers do not seem common. An additional benefit of hysterectomy is that it negates the increased risk of endometrial cancer[116,171] in those BRCA mutation carriers taking tamoxifen as adjuvant treatment of breast cancer, or as chemoprevention. Another consideration is that a rare form of endometrial cancer, uterine papillary serous endometrial cancer, has been identified in *BRCA* mutation carriers and hysterectomy removes this, albeit low, risk.[172,173] Although adding hysterectomy to RRSO increases the complexity, cost, and complication rate of the procedure, particularly in women with prior abdominal surgery, many women carrying BRCA mutations do select this option.[174]

Hormone replacement therapy

Combination hormone replacement therapy (HRT) has been shown to increase the risk of breast cancer in the general population when used long term in postmenopausal women. The studies showing this increased risk predominantly involved women who had undergone natural menopause and who were past their menopausal transition.[175] *BRCA* carriers who elect RRSO by age 40 years (according to the NCCN recommendations) experience surgical menopause an average of 10 years earlier than natural menopause, and have an abrupt rather than gradual decline in hormones that may result in substantial menopausal symptoms, including hot flashes, vaginal dryness, and changes in sexual function.[160] In addition, these women experience rapid bone loss associated with the loss of estrogen. Because *BRCA* carriers are at increased risk of breast cancer, these women may be concerned about using hormones to prevent or treat these symptoms (Case Study 4). Several studies have evaluated the risk of breast cancer with the use of post-RRSO HRT.[151,176] In the landmark study by Rebbeck and colleagues[151] in 2005, short-term use (up to 3.6 years) of HRT in *BRCA1/2* carriers did not increase the risk of breast cancer, which had already been reduced by oophorectomy.

Case Study 4. HRT after salpingo-oophorectomy

A 37-year-old G4P4 *BRCA1* carrier presents to her physician to discuss prophylactic bilateral salpingo-oophorectomy. She has completed childbearing, already had a bilateral PM with reconstruction, but has been reluctant to remove her ovaries because of concerns about menopausal symptoms. She would like to discuss her options for HRT and her residual breast cancer risk. After the different surgical options and risks are presented to the patient, she elects to have a laparoscopic salpingo-oophorectomy/hysterectomy and she is placed on estrogen replacement therapy after surgery.

Key points: HRT alleviates symptoms of menopause in young *BRCA* carriers who undergo bilateral salpingo-oophorectomy and is considered an option until the natural age of menopause. If a hysterectomy is performed at the time of RRSO, combined hormone therapy is not necessary and estrogen-only therapy is indicated.

Chemoprevention with OCPs

Although controversial in terms of impact on breast cancer risk, there is substantial evidence that oral contraceptives have a duration-dependent protective effect on rates of ovarian cancer.[81,177,178] This effect has been shown in the general population[179–181] as well as in *BRCA* mutation carriers.[177,179,182,183] The estimated risk reduction for carriers is 33% to 38% after 5 years of use.[177,182] On average, each year of use confers a 5% to 13% protective benefit.[177,182]

Other Gynecologic Surgery

Early fallopian tube cancers have been discovered at the time of RRSO, leading researchers to think that surgical removal of the fallopian tube and, in particular, the fimbria, may confer some protective benefit for *BRCA* mutation carriers.[184] Studies are ongoing to test this hypothesis.[185] However, given that hormonal function would be retained, the risks of hormone-sensitive breast cancer are unlikely to be mitigated with salpingectomy alone. At present, there are not enough data to recommend routine salpingectomy in young women with *BRCA* mutations who wish to retain their ovarian function.

Other related cancer risks

BRCA mutation carriers are at increased risk for other cancers, albeit to a lesser degree than the highly penetrant breast and ovarian/fallopian tube/peritoneal cancers. As described earlier, male *BRCA1* mutation carriers are at increased risk for breast cancer,[186–188] but also for prostate cancer,[189,190] and for both men and women there seems to be an increased risk of pancreatic cancer,[191–193] although the age of onset seems similar to that of sporadic cancer.[190,192,193] *BRCA2* mutation carriers have been shown to have even higher risks of male breast cancer,[67,188,194,195] pancreatic cancer,[196,197] and prostate cancer,[189,191,198,199] and prostate cancer tends to be of earlier onset than sporadic cancer.[191,200] Melanoma is also considered part of the *BRCA2* spectrum, although the relative risks are low compared with other malignancies.[186,191,200]

To date, pancreatic cancer screening outside a clinical research trial is not generally recommended for *BRCA* mutation carriers. In terms of melanoma, annual dermatologic[22] and ocular examinations are recommended,[186] and standard sun protection measures should also be encouraged.

SUMMARY

Although there is now a substantial body of knowledge regarding the efficacy of cancer risk assessment, genetic counseling and testing, and medical management for HBOC, many women who may carry a *BRCA1/2* mutation remain unidentified. As primary care givers for women, a clear understanding of the diagnosis and clinical management of HBOC is essential for obstetricians/gynecologists and other women's health practitioners. Based on family history, it is possible to identify women at risk of carrying a *BRCA1/2* mutation, allowing for cancer risk assessment, appropriate genetic testing, and initiation of screening and prevention strategies before a diagnosis of cancer occurs. Evidence-based management strategies have been shown to reduce cancer incidence in *BRCA* mutation carriers, and also to improve overall survival. In addition, improvements in breast cancer diagnostic methods, treatment, and prophylactic strategies have resulted in higher survival rates for women with HBOC affected by breast cancer. These women and those who remain cancer free present for routine gynecologic care faced with complex issues. Women's health providers with a strong working knowledge of HBOC must ensure that they stay up to date with emerging data and available resources to provide appropriate care to women and families affected by *BRCA1/2* mutations.

REFERENCES

1. Siegel R, Naishadham D, Jemal A. Cancer statistics, 2013. CA Cancer J Clin 2013;63(1):11–30.
2. Claus EB, Schildkraut JM, Thompson WD, et al. The genetic attributable risk of breast and ovarian cancer. Cancer 1996;77(11):2318–24.
3. Rubinstein W. The genetics of breast cancer. Malden (MA): Blackwell Science; 2001.
4. Weissman SM, Weiss SM, Newlin AC. Genetic testing by cancer site: ovary. Cancer J 2012;18(4):320–7.
5. Kurian AW. BRCA1 and BRCA2 mutations across race and ethnicity: distribution and clinical implications. Curr Opin Obstet Gynecol 2010;22(1):72–8.
6. Pal T, Permuth-Wey J, Betts JA, et al. BRCA1 and BRCA2 mutations account for a large proportion of ovarian carcinoma cases. Cancer 2005;104(12):2807–16.
7. Risch HA, McLaughlin JR, Cole DE, et al. Population BRCA1 and BRCA2 mutation frequencies and cancer penetrances: a kin-cohort study in Ontario, Canada. J Natl Cancer Inst 2006;98(23):1694–706.
8. Group ABCS. Prevalence and penetrance of BRCA1 and BRCA2 mutations in a population-based series of breast cancer cases. Anglian Breast Cancer Study Group. Br J Cancer 2000;83(10):1301–8.
9. Miki Y, Swensen J, Shattuck-Eidens D, et al. A strong candidate for the breast and ovarian cancer susceptibility gene BRCA1. Science 1994;266(5182):66–71.
10. Wooster R, Bignell G, Lancaster J, et al. Identification of the breast cancer susceptibility gene BRCA2. Nature 1995;378(6559):789–92.
11. Nelson HD, Huffman LH, Fu R, et al. Genetic risk assessment and BRCA mutation testing for breast and ovarian cancer susceptibility: systematic evidence review for the U.S. Preventive Services Task Force. Ann Intern Med 2005;143(5):362–79.
12. Risch HA, McLaughlin JR, Cole DE, et al. Prevalence and penetrance of germline BRCA1 and BRCA2 mutations in a population series of 649 women with ovarian cancer. Am J Hum Genet 2001;68(3):700–10.
13. Roa BB, Boyd AA, Volcik K, et al. Ashkenazi Jewish population frequencies for common mutations in BRCA1 and BRCA2. Nat Genet 1996;14(2):185–7.
14. Callahan MJ, Crum CP, Medeiros F, et al. Primary fallopian tube malignancies in BRCA-positive women undergoing surgery for ovarian cancer risk reduction. J Clin Oncol 2007;25(25):3985–90.
15. Medeiros F, Muto MG, Lee Y, et al. The tubal fimbria is a preferred site for early adenocarcinoma in women with familial ovarian cancer syndrome. Am J Surg Pathol 2006;30(2):230–6.

16. Vicus D, Finch A, Cass I, et al. Prevalence of BRCA1 and BRCA2 germ line mutations among women with carcinoma of the fallopian tube. Gynecol Oncol 2010;118(3):299–302.

17. Reitsma W, de Bock GH, Oosterwijk JC, et al. Support of the 'fallopian tube hypothesis' in a prospective series of risk-reducing salpingo-oophorectomy specimens. Eur J Cancer 2013;49(1):132–41.

18. Chen S, Parmigiani G. Meta-analysis of BRCA1 and BRCA2 penetrance. J Clin Oncol 2007;25(11):1329–33.

19. U.S. Preventive Services Task Force. Genetic risk assessment and BRCA mutation testing for breast and ovarian cancer susceptibility: recommendation statement. Ann Intern Med 2005;143(5):355–61.

20. American College of Obstetricians and Gynecologists, ACOG Committee on Practice Bulletins–Gynecology, ACOG Committee on Genetics, Society of Gynecologic Oncologists. ACOG Practice Bulletin No. 103: hereditary breast and ovarian cancer syndrome. Obstet Gynecol 2009;113(4): 957–66.

21. Lancaster JM, Powell CB, Kauff ND, et al. Society of Gynecologic Oncologists Education Committee statement on risk assessment for inherited gynecologic cancer predispositions. Gynecol Oncol 2007;107(2):159–62.

22. National Comprehensive Cancer Network. Clinical practice guidelines in oncology. Genetic/familial high-risk assessment: breast and ovarian. 2013. Available at: http://www.nccn.org/professionals/physician_gls/pdf/genetics_screening.pdf. Accessed March 1, 2013.

23. Hoskins KF, Zwaagstra A, Ranz M. Validation of a tool for identifying women at high risk for hereditary breast cancer in population-based screening. Cancer 2006;107(8):1769–76.

24. Teller P, Hoskins KF, Zwaagstra A, et al. Validation of the pedigree assessment tool (PAT) in families with BRCA1 and BRCA2 mutations. Ann Surg Oncol 2010; 17(1):240–6.

25. Bellcross C. Further development and evaluation of a breast/ovarian cancer genetics referral screening tool. Genet Med 2010;12(4):240.

26. Bellcross CA, Lemke AA, Pape LS, et al. Evaluation of a breast/ovarian cancer genetics referral screening tool in a mammography population. Genet Med 2009;11(11):783–9.

27. Gail MH, Brinton LA, Byar DP, et al. Projecting individualized probabilities of developing breast cancer for white females who are being examined annually. J Natl Cancer Inst 1989;81(24):1879–86.

28. Cancer Co. Cancer Program Standards 2012: ensuring patient-centered care. 2012; V1.1. Available at: http://www.facs.org/cancer/coc/programstandards2012. pdf. Accessed March 1, 2012.

29. Berliner JL, Fay AM, Cummings SA, et al. NSGC practice guideline: risk assessment and genetic counseling for hereditary breast and ovarian cancer. J Genet Couns 2013;22(2):155–63.

30. Riley BD, Culver JO, Skrzynia C, et al. Essential elements of genetic cancer risk assessment, counseling, and testing: updated recommendations of the National Society of Genetic Counselors. J Genet Couns 2012;21(2):151–61.

31. Robson ME, Storm CD, Weitzel J, et al. American Society of Clinical Oncology policy statement update: genetic and genomic testing for cancer susceptibility. J Clin Oncol 2010;28(5):893–901.

32. Matloff ET, Brierley KL. The double-helix derailed: the story of the BRCA patent. Lancet 2010;376(9738):314–5.

33. Domchek SM, Gaudet MM, Stopfer JE, et al. Breast cancer risks in individuals testing negative for a known family mutation in BRCA1 or BRCA2. Breast Cancer Res Treat 2010;119(2):409–14.
34. Kauff ND, Mitra N, Robson ME, et al. Risk of ovarian cancer in BRCA1 and BRCA2 mutation-negative hereditary breast cancer families. J Natl Cancer Inst 2005;97(18):1382–4.
35. Petrucelli N, Daly MB, Feldman GL. Hereditary breast and ovarian cancer due to mutations in BRCA1 and BRCA2. Genet Med 2010;12(5):245–59.
36. Shannon KM, Chittenden A. Genetic testing by cancer site: breast. Cancer J 2012;18(4):310–9.
37. Weitzel JN, Blazer KR, Macdonald DJ, et al. Genetics, genomics, and cancer risk assessment: State of the Art and Future Directions in the Era of Personalized Medicine. CA Cancer J Clin 2011;61:327–59.
38. Shuen AY, Foulkes WD. Inherited mutations in breast cancer genes–risk and response. J Mammary Gland Biol Neoplasia 2011;16(1):3–15.
39. Eng C, Sharp RR. Bioethical and clinical dilemmas of direct-to-consumer personal genomic testing: the problem of misattributed equivalence. Sci Transl Med 2010;2(17):1–5.
40. Wacholder S, Hartge P, Prentice R, et al. Performance of common genetic variants in breast-cancer risk models. N Engl J Med 2010;362(11):986–93.
41. Brandt A, Bermejo JL, Sundquist J, et al. Age of onset in familial cancer. Ann Oncol 2008;19(12):2084–8.
42. Forman AD, Hall MJ. Influence of race/ethnicity on genetic counseling and testing for hereditary breast and ovarian cancer. Breast J 2009;15(Suppl 1):S56–62.
43. Kieran S, Loescher LJ, Lim KH. The role of financial factors in acceptance of clinical BRCA genetic testing. Genet Test 2007;11(1):101–10.
44. Lowstuter KJ, Sand S, Blazer KR, et al. Influence of genetic discrimination perceptions and knowledge on cancer genetics referral practice among clinicians. Genet Med 2008;10(9):691–8.
45. Centers for Disease Control and Prevention. Health plan implementation of U.S. Preventive Services Task Force A and B recommendations–Colorado, 2010. MMWR Morb Mortal Wkly Rep 2011;60(39):1348–50.
46. Institute NHGR. Genetic discrimination. Available at: http://www.genome.gov/10002077. Accessed March 1, 2013.
47. Hall JP, Moore JM. The Affordable Care Act's pre-existing condition insurance plan: enrollment, costs, and lessons for reform. Issue Brief (Commonw Fund) 2012;24:1–13.
48. Hamilton JG, Lobel M, Moyer A. Emotional distress following genetic testing for hereditary breast and ovarian cancer: a meta-analytic review. Health Psychol 2009;28(4):510–8.
49. Lerman C, Hughes C, Lemon SJ, et al. What you don't know can hurt you: adverse psychologic effects in members of BRCA1-linked and BRCA2-linked families who decline genetic testing. J Clin Oncol 1998;16(5):1650–4.
50. Lynch HT, Snyder C, Lynch JF, et al. Patient responses to the disclosure of BRCA mutation tests in hereditary breast-ovarian cancer families. Cancer Genet Cytogenet 2006;165(2):91–7.
51. Litton JK, Ready K, Chen H, et al. Earlier age of onset of BRCA mutation-related cancers in subsequent generations. Cancer 2012;118(2):321–5.
52. Easton DF, Ford D, Bishop DT. Breast and ovarian cancer incidence in BRCA1-mutation carriers. Breast Cancer Linkage Consortium. Am J Hum Genet 1995;56(1):265–71.

53. Ford D, Easton DF, Stratton M, et al. Genetic heterogeneity and penetrance analysis of the BRCA1 and BRCA2 genes in breast cancer families. The Breast Cancer Linkage Consortium. Am J Hum Genet 1998;62(3):676–89.

54. Antoniou A, Pharoah PD, Narod S, et al. Average risks of breast and ovarian cancer associated with BRCA1 or BRCA2 mutations detected in case series unselected for family history: a combined analysis of 22 studies. Am J Hum Genet 2003;72(5):1117–30.

55. Hamilton R, Hurley KE. Conditions and consequences of a BRCA mutation in young, single women of childbearing age. Oncol Nurs Forum 2010;37(5): 627–34.

56. Evans DG, Lalloo F, Ashcroft L, et al. Uptake of risk-reducing surgery in unaffected women at high risk of breast and ovarian cancer is risk, age, and time dependent. Cancer Epidemiol Biomarkers Prev 2009;18(8):2318–24.

57. Donnelly LS, Watson M, Moynihan C, et al. Reproductive decision-making in young female carriers of a BRCA mutation. Hum Reprod 2013;28(4):1006–12.

58. Sigal BM, Munoz DF, Kurian AW, et al. A simulation model to predict the impact of prophylactic surgery and screening on the life expectancy of BRCA1 and BRCA2 mutation carriers. Cancer Epidemiol Biomarkers Prev 2012;21(7): 1066–77.

59. Schackmann EA, Munoz DF, Mills MA, et al. Feasibility evaluation of an online tool to guide decisions for BRCA1/2 mutation carriers. Fam Cancer 2013; 12(1):65–73.

60. Brose MS, Rebbeck TR, Calzone KA, et al. Cancer risk estimates for BRCA1 mutation carriers identified in a risk evaluation program. J Natl Cancer Inst 2002;94(18):1365–72.

61. Metcalfe K, Lynch HT, Ghadirian P, et al. Contralateral breast cancer in BRCA1 and BRCA2 mutation carriers. J Clin Oncol 2004;22(12):2328–35.

62. Tung N. Management of women with BRCA mutations: a 41-year-old woman with a BRCA mutation and a recent history of breast cancer. JAMA 2011;305(21): 2211–20.

63. Stucky CC, Gray RJ, Wasif N, et al. Increase in contralateral prophylactic mastectomy: echoes of a bygone era? Surgical trends for unilateral breast cancer. Ann Surg Oncol 2010;17(Suppl 3):330–7.

64. Verhoog LC, Brekelmans CT, Seynaeve C, et al. Contralateral breast cancer risk is influenced by the age at onset in BRCA1-associated breast cancer. Br J Cancer 2000;83(3):384–6.

65. Pierce LJ, Haffty BG. Radiotherapy in the treatment of hereditary breast cancer. Semin Radiat Oncol 2011;21(1):43–50.

66. Reding KW, Bernstein JL, Langholz BM, et al. Adjuvant systemic therapy for breast cancer in BRCA1/BRCA2 mutation carriers in a population-based study of risk of contralateral breast cancer. Breast Cancer Res Treat 2010;123(2): 491–8.

67. Thompson D, Easton D. Variation in cancer risks, by mutation position, in BRCA2 mutation carriers. Am J Hum Genet 2001;68(2):410–9.

68. Giordano SH, Cohen DS, Buzdar AU, et al. Breast carcinoma in men: a population-based study. Cancer 2004;101(1):51–7.

69. Levy-Lahad E, Friedman E. Cancer risks among BRCA1 and BRCA2 mutation carriers. Br J Cancer 2007;96(1):11–5.

70. Simchoni S, Friedman E, Kaufman B, et al. Familial clustering of site-specific cancer risks associated with BRCA1 and BRCA2 mutations in the Ashkenazi Jewish population. Proc Natl Acad Sci U S A 2006;103(10):3770–4.

71. Antoniou AC, Sinilnikova OM, Simard J, et al. RAD51 135G->C modifies breast cancer risk among BRCA2 mutation carriers: results from a combined analysis of 19 studies. Am J Hum Genet 2007;81(6):1186–200.

72. Metcalfe K, Lubinski J, Lynch HT, et al. Family history of cancer and cancer risks in women with BRCA1 or BRCA2 mutations. J Natl Cancer Inst 2010;102(24): 1874–8.

73. Kotsopoulos J, Lubinski J, Lynch HT, et al. Age at menarche and the risk of breast cancer in BRCA1 and BRCA2 mutation carriers. Cancer Causes Control 2005;16(6):667–74.

74. Nedelcu R, Liede A, Aube J, et al. BRCA mutations in Italian breast/ovarian cancer families. Eur J Hum Genet 2002;10(2):150–2.

75. Cullinane CA, Lubinski J, Neuhausen SL, et al. Effect of pregnancy as a risk factor for breast cancer in BRCA1/BRCA2 mutation carriers. Int J Cancer 2005; 117(6):988–91.

76. Kotsopoulos J, Lubinski J, Salmena L, et al. Breastfeeding and the risk of breast cancer in BRCA1 and BRCA2 mutation carriers. Breast Cancer Res 2012;14(2):R42.

77. Antoniou AC, Rookus M, Andrieu N, et al. Reproductive and hormonal factors, and ovarian cancer risk for BRCA1 and BRCA2 mutation carriers: results from the International BRCA1/2 Carrier Cohort Study. Cancer Epidemiol Biomarkers Prev 2009;18(2):601–10.

78. Andrieu N, Goldgar DE, Easton DF, et al. Pregnancies, breast-feeding, and breast cancer risk in the International BRCA1/2 Carrier Cohort Study (IBCCS). J Natl Cancer Inst 2006;98(8):535–44.

79. King MC, Marks JH, Mandell JB. Breast and ovarian cancer risks due to inherited mutations in BRCA1 and BRCA2. Science 2003;302(5645):643–6.

80. Kotsopoulos J, Olopado OI, Ghadirian P, et al. Changes in body weight and the risk of breast cancer in BRCA1 and BRCA2 mutation carriers. Breast Cancer Res 2005;7(5):R833–43.

81. Cibula D, Zikan M, Dusek L, et al. Oral contraceptives and risk of ovarian and breast cancers in BRCA mutation carriers: a meta-analysis. Expert Rev Anticancer Ther 2011;11(8):1197–207.

82. Iodice S, Barile M, Rotmensz N, et al. Oral contraceptive use and breast or ovarian cancer risk in BRCA1/2 carriers: a meta-analysis. Eur J Cancer 2010; 46(12):2275–84.

83. Robson ME, Chappuis PO, Satagopan J, et al. A combined analysis of outcome following breast cancer: differences in survival based on BRCA1/BRCA2 mutation status and administration of adjuvant treatment. Breast Cancer Res 2004; 6(1):R8–17.

84. Rennert G, Bisland-Naggan S, Barnett-Griness O, et al. Clinical outcomes of breast cancer in carriers of BRCA1 and BRCA2 mutations. N Engl J Med 2007;357(2):115–23.

85. Brekelmans CT, Tilanus-Linthorst MM, Seynaeve C, et al. Tumour characteristics, survival and prognostic factors of hereditary breast cancer from BRCA2-, BRCA1- and non-BRCA1/2 families as compared to sporadic breast cancer cases. Eur J Cancer 2007;43(5):867–76.

86. Bordeleau L, Panchal S, Goodwin P. Prognosis of BRCA-associated breast cancer: a summary of evidence. Breast Cancer Res Treat 2010;119(1):13–24.

87. Mavaddat N, Barrowdale D, Andrulis IL, et al. Pathology of breast and ovarian cancers among BRCA1 and BRCA2 mutation carriers: results from the Consortium of Investigators of Modifiers of BRCA1/2 (CIMBA). Cancer Epidemiol Biomarkers Prev 2012;21(1):134–47.

88. Lakhani SR, Van De Vijver MJ, Jacquemier J, et al. The pathology of familial breast cancer: predictive value of immunohistochemical markers estrogen receptor, progesterone receptor, HER-2, and p53 in patients with mutations in BRCA1 and BRCA2. J Clin Oncol 2002;20(9):2310–8.

89. Lakhani SR, Reis-Filho JS, Fulford L, et al. Prediction of BRCA1 status in patients with breast cancer using estrogen receptor and basal phenotype. Clin Cancer Res 2005;11(14):5175–80.

90. Wevers MR, Hahn DE, Verhoef S, et al. Breast cancer genetic counseling after diagnosis but before treatment: a pilot study on treatment consequences and psychological impact. Patient Educ Couns 2012;89(1):89–95.

91. Chung A, Huynh K, Lawrence C, et al. Comparison of patient characteristics and outcomes of contralateral prophylactic mastectomy and unilateral total mastectomy in breast cancer patients. Ann Surg Oncol 2012;19(8):2600–6.

92. Pierce LJ, Phillips KA, Griffith KA, et al. Local therapy in BRCA1 and BRCA2 mutation carriers with operable breast cancer: comparison of breast conservation and mastectomy. Breast Cancer Res Treat 2010;121(2):389–98.

93. Heemskerk-Gerritsen BA, Kriege M, Seynaeve C. Association of risk-reducing surgery with cancer risks and mortality in BRCA mutation carriers. JAMA 2010;304(24):2695 [author reply: 2695–6].

94. van Sprundel TC, Schmidt MK, Rookus MA, et al. Risk reduction of contralateral breast cancer and survival after contralateral prophylactic mastectomy in BRCA1 or BRCA2 mutation carriers. Br J Cancer 2005;93(3):287–92.

95. Kriege M, Seynaeve C, Meijers-Heijboer H, et al. Sensitivity to first-line chemotherapy for metastatic breast cancer in BRCA1 and BRCA2 mutation carriers. J Clin Oncol 2009;27(23):3764–71.

96. Tutt A, Robson M, Garber JE, et al. Oral poly(ADP-ribose) polymerase inhibitor olaparib in patients with BRCA1 or BRCA2 mutations and advanced breast cancer: a proof-of-concept trial. Lancet 2010;376(9737):235–44.

97. Warner E, Plewes DB, Hill KA, et al. Surveillance of BRCA1 and BRCA2 mutation carriers with magnetic resonance imaging, ultrasound, mammography, and clinical breast examination. JAMA 2004;292(11):1317–25.

98. Kuhl CK, Schrading S, Leutner CC, et al. Mammography, breast ultrasound, and magnetic resonance imaging for surveillance of women at high familial risk for breast cancer. J Clin Oncol 2005;23(33):8469–76.

99. Lowry KP, Lee JM, Kong CY, et al. Annual screening strategies in BRCA1 and BRCA2 gene mutation carriers: a comparative effectiveness analysis. Cancer 2012;118(8):2021–30.

100. Saslow D, Boetes C, Burke W, et al. American Cancer Society guidelines for breast screening with MRI as an adjunct to mammography. CA Cancer J Clin 2007;57(2):75–89.

101. Warner E, Hill K, Causer P, et al. Prospective study of breast cancer incidence in women with a BRCA1 or BRCA2 mutation under surveillance with and without magnetic resonance imaging. J Clin Oncol 2011;29(13):1664–9.

102. Cott Chubiz JE, Lee JM, Gilmore ME, et al. Cost-effectiveness of alternating magnetic resonance imaging and digital mammography screening in BRCA1 and BRCA2 gene mutation carriers. Cancer 2013;119(6):1266–76.

103. Kriege M, Brekelmans CT, Boetes C, et al. Efficacy of MRI and mammography for breast-cancer screening in women with a familial or genetic predisposition. N Engl J Med 2004;351(5):427–37.

104. Leach MO, Boggis CR, Dixon AK, et al. Screening with magnetic resonance imaging and mammography of a UK population at high familial risk of breast

cancer: a prospective multicentre cohort study (MARIBS). Lancet 2005; 365(9473):1769–78.

105. Kriege M, Brekelmans CT, Obdeijn IM, et al. Factors affecting sensitivity and specificity of screening mammography and MRI in women with an inherited risk for breast cancer. Breast Cancer Res Treat 2006;100(1):109–19.

106. Passaperuma K, Warner E, Causer PA, et al. Long-term results of screening with magnetic resonance imaging in women with BRCA mutations. Br J Cancer 2012; 107(1):24–30.

107. Robson M, Offit K. Clinical practice. Management of an inherited predisposition to breast cancer. N Engl J Med 2007;357(2):154–62.

108. Domchek SM, Friebel TM, Singer CF, et al. Association of risk-reducing surgery in BRCA1 or BRCA2 mutation carriers with cancer risk and mortality. JAMA 2010;304(9):967–75.

109. Hartmann LC, Sellers TA, Schaid DJ, et al. Efficacy of bilateral prophylactic mastectomy in BRCA1 and BRCA2 gene mutation carriers. J Natl Cancer Inst 2001; 93(21):1633–7.

110. Meijers-Heijboer H, van Geel B, van Putten WL, et al. Breast cancer after prophylactic bilateral mastectomy in women with a BRCA1 or BRCA2 mutation. N Engl J Med 2001;345(3):159–64.

111. Rebbeck TR, Friebel T, Lynch HT, et al. Bilateral prophylactic mastectomy reduces breast cancer risk in BRCA1 and BRCA2 mutation carriers: the PROSE Study Group. J Clin Oncol 2004;22(6):1055–62.

112. Metcalfe KA, Birenbaum-Carmeli D, Lubinski J, et al. International variation in rates of uptake of preventive options in BRCA1 and BRCA2 mutation carriers. Int J Cancer 2008;122(9):2017–22.

113. Eisen A, Lubinski J, Klijn J, et al. Breast cancer risk following bilateral oophorectomy in BRCA1 and BRCA2 mutation carriers: an international case-control study. J Clin Oncol 2005;23(30):7491–6.

114. Kauff ND, Domchek SM, Friebel TM, et al. Risk-reducing salpingo-oophorectomy for the prevention of BRCA1- and BRCA2-associated breast and gynecologic cancer: a multicenter, prospective study. J Clin Oncol 2008; 26(8):1331–7.

115. Rebbeck TR, Kauff ND, Domchek SM. Meta-analysis of risk reduction estimates associated with risk-reducing salpingo-oophorectomy in BRCA1 or BRCA2 mutation carriers. J Natl Cancer Inst 2009;101(2):80–7.

116. Fisher B, Costantino JP, Wickerham DL, et al. Tamoxifen for prevention of breast cancer: report of the National Surgical Adjuvant Breast and Bowel Project P-1 Study. J Natl Cancer Inst 1998;90(18):1371–88.

117. King MC, Wieand S, Hale K, et al. Tamoxifen and breast cancer incidence among women with inherited mutations in BRCA1 and BRCA2: National Surgical Adjuvant Breast and Bowel Project (NSABP-P1) Breast Cancer Prevention Trial. JAMA 2001;286(18):2251–6.

118. Gronwald J, Tung N, Foulkes WD, et al. Tamoxifen and contralateral breast cancer in BRCA1 and BRCA2 carriers: an update. Int J Cancer 2006;118(9):2281–4.

119. Metcalfe KA, Snyder C, Seidel J, et al. The use of preventive measures among healthy women who carry a BRCA1 or BRCA2 mutation. Fam Cancer 2005;4(2): 97–103.

120. Uray IP, Brown PH. Chemoprevention of hormone receptor-negative breast cancer: new approaches needed. Recent Results Cancer Res 2011;188:147–62.

121. Long KC, Kauff ND. Hereditary ovarian cancer: recent molecular insights and their impact on screening strategies. Curr Opin Oncol 2011;23(5):526–30.

122. Levine DA, Argenta PA, Yee CJ, et al. Fallopian tube and primary peritoneal carcinomas associated with BRCA mutations. J Clin Oncol 2003;21(22):4222–7.

123. Piver MS, Jishi MF, Tsukada Y, et al. Primary peritoneal carcinoma after prophylactic oophorectomy in women with a family history of ovarian cancer. A report of the Gilda Radner Familial Ovarian Cancer Registry. Cancer 1993; 71(9):2751–5.

124. Evans DG, Gaarenstroom KN, Stirling D, et al. Screening for familial ovarian cancer: poor survival of BRCA1/2 related cancers. J Med Genet 2009;46(9): 593–7.

125. Dann RB, Kelley JL, Zorn KK. Strategies for ovarian cancer prevention. Obstet Gynecol Clin North Am 2007;34(4):667–86.

126. Lakhani SR, Manek S, Penault-Llorca F, et al. Pathology of ovarian cancers in BRCA1 and BRCA2 carriers. Clin Cancer Res 2004;10(7):2473–81.

127. Berchuck A, Heron KA, Carney ME, et al. Frequency of germline and somatic BRCA1 mutations in ovarian cancer. Clin Cancer Res 1998;4(10):2433–7.

128. Powell CB, Kenley E, Chen LM, et al. Risk-reducing salpingo-oophorectomy in BRCA mutation carriers: role of serial sectioning in the detection of occult malignancy. J Clin Oncol 2005;23(1):127–32.

129. Shaw PA, Rouzbahman M, Pizer ES, et al. Candidate serous cancer precursors in fallopian tube epithelium of BRCA1/2 mutation carriers. Mod Pathol 2009; 22(9):1133–8.

130. Aziz S, Kuperstein G, Rosen B, et al. A genetic epidemiological study of carcinoma of the fallopian tube. Gynecol Oncol 2001;80(3):341–5.

131. Boyd J, Sonoda Y, Federici MG, et al. Clinicopathologic features of BRCA-linked and sporadic ovarian cancer. JAMA 2000;283(17):2260–5.

132. Bolton KL, Chenevix-Trench G, Goh C, et al. Association between BRCA1 and BRCA2 mutations and survival in women with invasive epithelial ovarian cancer. JAMA 2012;307(4):382–90.

133. Cass I, Baldwin RL, Varkey T, et al. Improved survival in women with BRCA-associated ovarian carcinoma. Cancer 2003;97(9):2187–95.

134. Lacour RA, Westin SN, Meyer LA, et al. Improved survival in non-Ashkenazi Jewish ovarian cancer patients with BRCA1 and BRCA2 gene mutations. Gynecol Oncol 2011;121(2):358–63.

135. Tan DS, Rothermundt C, Thomas K, et al. "BRCAness" syndrome in ovarian cancer: a case-control study describing the clinical features and outcome of patients with epithelial ovarian cancer associated with BRCA1 and BRCA2 mutations. J Clin Oncol 2008;26(34):5530–6.

136. Hyman DM, Zhou Q, Iasonos A, et al. Improved survival for BRCA2-associated serous ovarian cancer compared with both BRCA-negative and BRCA1-associated serous ovarian cancer. Cancer 2012;118(15):3703–9.

137. Liu G, Yang D, Sun Y, et al. Differing clinical impact of BRCA1 and BRCA2 mutations in serous ovarian cancer. Pharmacogenomics 2012;13(13):1523–35.

138. Fong PC, Yap TA, Boss DS, et al. Poly(ADP)-ribose polymerase inhibition: frequent durable responses in BRCA carrier ovarian cancer correlating with platinum-free interval. J Clin Oncol 2010;28(15):2512–9.

139. Fong PC, Boss DS, Yap TA, et al. Inhibition of poly(ADP-ribose) polymerase in tumors from BRCA mutation carriers. N Engl J Med 2009;361(2):123–34.

140. Pennington KP, Swisher EM. Hereditary ovarian cancer: beyond the usual suspects. Gynecol Oncol 2012;124(2):347–53.

141. Wilkinson-Ryan I, Mutch D. A review of iniparib in ovarian cancer. Expert Opin Investig Drugs 2013;22(3):399–405.

142. Ratner ES, Sartorelli AC, Lin ZP. Poly (ADP-ribose) polymerase inhibitors: on the horizon of tailored and personalized therapies for epithelial ovarian cancer. Curr Opin Oncol 2012;24(5):564–71.

143. Woodward ER, Sleightholme HV, Considine AM, et al. Annual surveillance by CA125 and transvaginal ultrasound for ovarian cancer in both high-risk and population risk women is ineffective. BJOG 2007;114(12):1500–9.

144. van der Velde NM, Mourits MJ, Arts HJ, et al. Time to stop ovarian cancer screening in BRCA1/2 mutation carriers? Int J Cancer 2009;124(4):919–23.

145. Clarke-Pearson DL. Clinical practice. Screening for ovarian cancer. N Engl J Med 2009;361(2):170–7.

146. Kauff ND, Satagopan JM, Robson ME, et al. Risk-reducing salpingo-oophorectomy in women with a BRCA1 or BRCA2 mutation. N Engl J Med 2002;346(21):1609–15.

147. Rhiem K, Foth D, Wappenschmidt B, et al. Risk-reducing salpingo-oophorectomy in BRCA1 and BRCA2 mutation carriers. Arch Gynecol Obstet 2011;283(3):623–7.

148. Kenkhuis MJ, de Bock GH, Elferink PO, et al. Short-term surgical outcome and safety of risk reducing salpingo-oophorectomy in BRCA1/2 mutation carriers. Maturitas 2010;66(3):310–4.

149. Lu KH, Garber JE, Cramer DW, et al. Occult ovarian tumors in women with BRCA1 or BRCA2 mutations undergoing prophylactic oophorectomy. J Clin Oncol 2000;18(14):2728–32.

150. Finch A, Beiner M, Lubinski J, et al. Salpingo-oophorectomy and the risk of ovarian, fallopian tube, and peritoneal cancers in women with a BRCA1 or BRCA2 mutation. JAMA 2006;296(2):185–92.

151. Rebbeck TR, Friebel T, Wagner T, et al. Effect of short-term hormone replacement therapy on breast cancer risk reduction after bilateral prophylactic oophorectomy in BRCA1 and BRCA2 mutation carriers: the PROSE Study Group. J Clin Oncol 2005;23(31):7804–10.

152. Leeper K, Garcia R, Swisher E, et al. Pathologic findings in prophylactic oophorectomy specimens in high-risk women. Gynecol Oncol 2002;87(1):52–6.

153. McLaughlin JR, Risch HA, Lubinski J, et al. Reproductive risk factors for ovarian cancer in carriers of BRCA1 or BRCA2 mutations: a case-control study. Lancet Oncol 2007;8(1):26–34.

154. Mingels MJ, Roelofsen T, van der Laak JA, et al. Tubal epithelial lesions in salpingo-oophorectomy specimens of BRCA-mutation carriers and controls. Gynecol Oncol 2012;127(1):88–93.

155. Agoff SN, Mendelin JE, Grieco VS, et al. Unexpected gynecologic neoplasms in patients with proven or suspected BRCA-1 or -2 mutations: implications for gross examination, cytology, and clinical follow-up. Am J Surg Pathol 2002; 26(2):171–8.

156. Landon G, Stewart J, Deavers M, et al. Peritoneal washing cytology in patients with BRCA1 or BRCA2 mutations undergoing risk-reducing salpingo-oophorectomies: a 10-year experience and reappraisal of its clinical utility. Gynecol Oncol 2012;125(3):683–6.

157. Rebbeck TR, Lynch HT, Neuhausen SL, et al. Prophylactic oophorectomy in carriers of BRCA1 or BRCA2 mutations. N Engl J Med 2002;346(21): 1616–22.

158. Finch A, Metcalfe KA, Chiang JK, et al. The impact of prophylactic salpingo-oophorectomy on menopausal symptoms and sexual function in women who carry a BRCA mutation. Gynecol Oncol 2011;121(1):163–8.

159. Finch A, Metcalfe KA, Chiang J, et al. The impact of prophylactic salpingo-oophorectomy on quality of life and psychological distress in women with a BRCA mutation. Psychooncology 2013;22(1):212–9.
160. Finch A, Evans G, Narod SA. BRCA carriers, prophylactic salpingo-oophorectomy and menopause: clinical management considerations and recommendations. Womens Health (Lond Engl) 2012;8(5):543–55.
161. Finch A, Narod SA. Quality of life and health status after prophylactic salpingo-oophorectomy in women who carry a BRCA mutation: a review. Maturitas 2011; 70(3):261–5.
162. Campfield Bonadies D, Moyer A, Matloff ET. What I wish I'd known before surgery: BRCA carriers' perspectives after bilateral salipingo-oophorectomy. Fam Cancer 2011;10(1):79–85.
163. Cohen JV, Chiel L, Boghossian L, et al. Non-cancer endpoints in BRCA1/2 carriers after risk-reducing salpingo-oophorectomy. Fam Cancer 2012;11(1):69–75.
164. Challberg J, Ashcroft L, Lalloo F, et al. Menopausal symptoms and bone health in women undertaking risk reducing bilateral salpingo-oophorectomy: significant bone health issues in those not taking HRT. Br J Cancer 2011;105(1):22–7.
165. Jacoby VL, Grady D, Wactawski-Wende J, et al. Oophorectomy vs ovarian conservation with hysterectomy: cardiovascular disease, hip fracture, and cancer in the Women's Health Initiative Observational Study. Arch Intern Med 2011;171(8): 760–8.
166. Vesco KK, Marshall LM, Nelson HD, et al. Surgical menopause and nonvertebral fracture risk among older US women. Menopause 2012;19(5):510–6.
167. Banks E, Reeves GK, Beral V, et al. Hip fracture incidence in relation to age, menopausal status, and age at menopause: prospective analysis. PLoS Med 2009;6(11):e1000181.
168. Rivera CM, Grossardt BR, Rhodes DJ, et al. Increased cardiovascular mortality after early bilateral oophorectomy. Menopause 2009;16(1):15–23.
169. Colditz GA, Willett WC, Stampfer MJ, et al. Menopause and the risk of coronary heart disease in women. N Engl J Med 1987;316(18):1105–10.
170. Atsma F, Bartelink ML, Grobbee DE, et al. Postmenopausal status and early menopause as independent risk factors for cardiovascular disease: a meta-analysis. Menopause 2006;13(2):265–79.
171. Beiner ME, Finch A, Rosen B, et al. The risk of endometrial cancer in women with BRCA1 and BRCA2 mutations. A prospective study. Gynecol Oncol 2007; 104(1):7–10.
172. Karlan BY, Baldwin RL, Lopez-Luevanos E, et al. Peritoneal serous papillary carcinoma, a phenotypic variant of familial ovarian cancer: implications for ovarian cancer screening. Am J Obstet Gynecol 1999;180(4):917–28.
173. Pennington KP, Walsh T, Lee M, et al. BRCA1, TP53, and CHEK2 germline mutations in uterine serous carcinoma. Cancer 2013;119(2):332–8.
174. Gabriel CA, Tigges-Cardwell J, Stopfer J, et al. Use of total abdominal hysterectomy and hormone replacement therapy in BRCA1 and BRCA2 mutation carriers undergoing risk-reducing salpingo-oophorectomy. Fam Cancer 2009; 8(1):23–8.
175. Chlebowski RT, Kuller LH, Prentice RL, et al. Breast cancer after use of estrogen plus progestin in postmenopausal women. N Engl J Med 2009;360(6):573–87.
176. Eisen A, Lubinski J, Gronwald J, et al. Hormone therapy and the risk of breast cancer in BRCA1 mutation carriers. J Natl Cancer Inst 2008;100(19):1361–7.
177. Narod SA, Sun P, Risch HA. Ovarian cancer, oral contraceptives, and BRCA mutations. N Engl J Med 2001;345(23):1706–7.

178. Gadducci A, Biglia N, Cosio S, et al. Gynaecologic challenging issues in the management of BRCA mutation carriers: oral contraceptives, prophylactic salpingo-oophorectomy and hormone replacement therapy. Gynecol Endocrinol 2010;26(8):568–77.

179. Rice LW. Hormone prevention strategies for breast, endometrial and ovarian cancers. Gynecol Oncol 2010;118(2):202–7.

180. Oral contraceptives cut inherited cancer risk. Contracept Technol Update 1998; 19(11):146–7.

181. Jensen JT, Speroff L. Health benefits of oral contraceptives. Obstet Gynecol Clin North Am 2000;27(4):705–21.

182. Whittemore AS, Balise RR, Pharoah PD, et al. Oral contraceptive use and ovarian cancer risk among carriers of BRCA1 or BRCA2 mutations. Br J Cancer 2004;91(11):1911–5.

183. Narod SA, Risch H, Moslehi R, et al. Oral contraceptives and the risk of hereditary ovarian cancer. Hereditary Ovarian Cancer Clinical Study Group. N Engl J Med 1998;339(7):424–8.

184. Kwon JS, Tinker A, Pansegrau G, et al. Prophylactic salpingectomy and delayed oophorectomy as an alternative for BRCA mutation carriers. Obstet Gynecol 2013;121(1):14–24.

185. Leblanc E, Narducci F, Farre I, et al. Radical fimbriectomy: a reasonable temporary risk-reducing surgery for selected women with a germ line mutation of BRCA 1 or 2 genes? Rationale and preliminary development. Gynecol Oncol 2011;121(3):472–6.

186. Liede A, Karlan BY, Narod SA. Cancer risks for male carriers of germline mutations in BRCA1 or BRCA2: a review of the literature. J Clin Oncol 2004;22(4): 735–42.

187. Friedman LS, Gayther SA, Kurosaki T, et al. Mutation analysis of BRCA1 and BRCA2 in a male breast cancer population. Am J Hum Genet 1997;60(2): 313–9.

188. Tai YC, Domchek S, Parmigiani G, et al. Breast cancer risk among male BRCA1 and BRCA2 mutation carriers. J Natl Cancer Inst 2007;99(23):1811–4.

189. Agalliu I, Gern R, Leanza S, et al. Associations of high-grade prostate cancer with BRCA1 and BRCA2 founder mutations. Clin Cancer Res 2009;15(3): 1112–20.

190. Cybulski C, Gorski B, Gronwald J, et al. BRCA1 mutations and prostate cancer in Poland. Eur J Cancer Prev 2008;17(1):62–6.

191. van Asperen CJ, Brohet RM, Meijers-Heijboer EJ, et al. Cancer risks in BRCA2 families: estimates for sites other than breast and ovary. J Med Genet 2005; 42(9):711–9.

192. Kim DH, Crawford B, Ziegler J, et al. Prevalence and characteristics of pancreatic cancer in families with BRCA1 and BRCA2 mutations. Fam Cancer 2009; 8(2):153–8.

193. Lynch HT, Deters CA, Snyder CL, et al. BRCA1 and pancreatic cancer: pedigree findings and their causal relationships. Cancer Genet Cytogenet 2005;158(2): 119–25.

194. Couch FJ, Farid LM, DeShano ML, et al. BRCA2 germline mutations in male breast cancer cases and breast cancer families. Nat Genet 1996;13(1):123–5.

195. Fentiman IS, Fourquet A, Hortobagyi GN. Male breast cancer. Lancet 2006; 367(9510):595–604.

196. Hahn SA, Greenhalf B, Ellis I, et al. BRCA2 germline mutations in familial pancreatic carcinoma. J Natl Cancer Inst 2003;95(3):214–21.

197. Murphy KM, Brune KA, Griffin C, et al. Evaluation of candidate genes MAP2K4, MADH4, ACVR1B, and BRCA2 in familial pancreatic cancer: deleterious BRCA2 mutations in 17%. Cancer Res 2002;62(13):3789–93.
198. Kirchhoff T, Kauff ND, Mitra N, et al. BRCA mutations and risk of prostate cancer in Ashkenazi Jews. Clin Cancer Res 2004;10(9):2918–21.
199. Ozcelik H, Schmocker B, Di Nicola N, et al. Germline BRCA2 6174delT mutations in Ashkenazi Jewish pancreatic cancer patients. Nat Genet 1997;16(1): 17–8.
200. Cancer risks in BRCA2 mutation carriers. The Breast Cancer Linkage Consortium. J Natl Cancer Inst 1999;91(15):1310–6.
201. Euhus DM, Robinson L. Genetic predisposition syndromes and their management. Surg Clin North Am 2013;93(2):341–62.

Health Disparities in Breast Cancer

Otis W. Brawley, MD

KEYWORDS

- Breast cancer • African American • Race • Mortality rate • Risk factor

KEY POINTS

- There has been a growing Black-White disparity in breast cancer mortality after a period of relative equivalence.
- Literature shows that Black Americans with breast cancer are less likely to receive optimal care compared with White Americans.
- Tumors in Black Americans are more likely to be poorly differentiated and estrogen receptor negative and exhibit a high S-phase fraction compared with tumors from White Americans.
- Differences in dietary habits, breast-feeding, and obesity account for some of the population differences in outcome among Black Americans.

Breast cancer is the most commonly diagnosed nonskin cancer and the second leading cause of cancer death among American women. In 2013, an estimated 232,000 American women will be diagnosed with invasive breast cancer and 39,600 will die from it. Breast cancer is also the most commonly diagnosed cancer and the second leading cause of cancer death among Black or African American (AA) women. It is estimated that 27,000 Black women will be diagnosed with invasive breast cancer in 2013 and slightly more than 6000 will die of it.[1]

The National Cancer Institute Surveillance, Epidemiology, and End Results (SEER) Program has published cancer data by race for more than 3 decades.[1] The data are approximately 3 years old when published. Age-adjusted incidence and mortality rates for the 5 racial/ethnic groups recognized by the US Census for 2005 to 2009 are listed in **Table 1**. The rates are age-adjusted to the year 2000 standard to remove the effect of the aging of the American population. Black and White Americans have higher breast cancer incidence and mortality rates compared with Asian, Hispanic, and Native Americans.

Disclosures: The author has nothing to disclose.
American Cancer Society, Emory University, 250 Williams Street, Atlanta, GA 30303, USA
E-mail address: otis.brawley@cancer.org

Table 1
NCI SEER annual incidence and mortality rates 100,000 population, averaging events in years 2005–2009

	Incidence	Mortality
All races	124.3	23.0
White	127.3	22.4
Black	121.2	31.6
Asian/Pacific	94.5	11.9
American Indian/Alaskan Native	80.6	16.6
Hispanic	92.7	14.9

Data are age-adjusted to the year 2000 standard.

These age-adjusted incidence and mortality rates can also be considered risk of breast cancer diagnosis and death. Age-adjusted incidence and mortality rates are the most accurate way to assess progress in the fight against breast cancer.[2]

The trend in age-adjusted incidence rate from 1975 to 2009 for Blacks and Whites is shown in **Fig. 1**. White women have consistently had higher incidence rates than Blacks. The increase in incidence from 1975 to 2000 is largely attributed to screening and awareness, although as discussed later, additional causes cannot be excluded and likely did contribute.

The trend in age-adjusted mortality from 1975 to 2009 for Black and White Americans is shown in **Fig. 2**. Of note, the age-adjusted mortality was essentially the same in the 1970s despite the higher incidence rate for Whites. There has been a 35% decrease in mortality among White Americans and a nearly 20% decline among Blacks.

Fig. 3 illustrates the age-specific incidence and mortality rates for Blacks and Whites during the period 2005 to 2009. Black women have higher age-specific mortality beginning in the third decade.

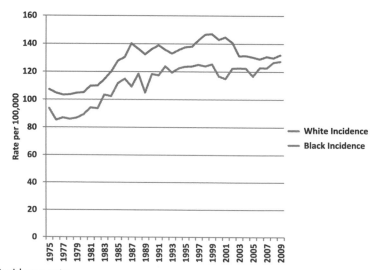

Fig. 1. Incidence rate.

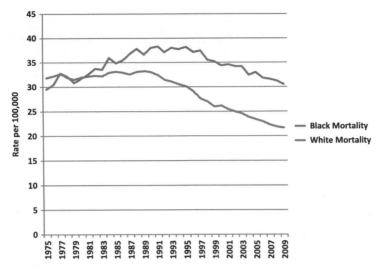

Fig. 2. Mortality rate.

The NCI SEER program collects stage in 3 categories: local, which roughly correlates with American Joint Committee on Cancer (AJCC) stage 1 and 2; regional, which approximates AJCC stage 3; and distant, which is AJCC stage 4. The Black-White difference in stage at diagnosis for those diagnosed during the period 2002 to 2008 is shown in **Table 2**. A higher proportion of Black women present with regional and distant disease (see **Table 2**).

Five-year survival rates by stage at diagnosis are shown in **Table 3**. There is a Black-White disparity, but survival figures are often misused or misinterpreted and should be used with caution.[2]

There has been much study to determine why Black women have higher mortality compared with Whites. This work has focused on the possibility of Blacks tending to have more aggressive breast cancer pathologic condition and less access to quality

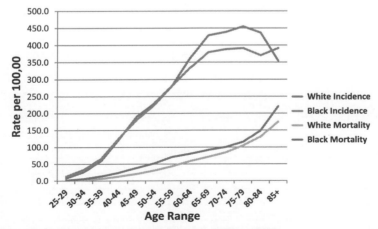

Fig. 3. Age-specific incidence and mortality rates 2005 to 2009.

Table 2
Breast cancer stage at diagnosis for Black and White Americans diagnosed in NCI SEER registries from 2002 to 2008

	Breast Cancer Stage at Diagnosis by Race	
SEER Stage	White	Black
Localized	61%	51%
Regional	32%	38%
Distant	5%	8%
Unstaged	2%	2%

care. Both are true. Tumors in Black Americans are more likely to be poorly differentiated and estrogen receptor negative and exhibit a high S-phase fraction compared with tumors from White Americans.

BREAST CANCER RISK FACTORS

Besides being female, increasing age is the most important risk factor for breast cancer. Some of the known modifiable risk factors for this disease include weight gain after age 18, being obese, physical inactivity, use of menopausal hormone therapy (estrogen and progestin), smoking, and alcohol consumption. Other risk factors, including having high breast density as seen on mammogram and high bone mineral density, are also correlated with an increased risk of breast cancer. Reproductive factors that increase risk include a long menstrual history, meaning menstruation beginning at an early age or associated with late menopause.[3]

There are several racial differences in the prevalence of risk factors. Approximately 50% of Black American women are obese, which compares to 35% of White women being obese.[4] Obesity is associated with increased risk of postmenopausal breast cancer and may be a cause of premenopausal disease.[5] Obese women are also more commonly diagnosed in advanced stages.[3] Physical inactivity is also common among Black women and possibly more common than among White women.[5]

Some older literature showed a correlation of increased consumption of dietary fat and increased risk of breast cancer. Evidence to support this dietary hypothesis has weakened over the past few years in favor of the theory that increased caloric intake and decreased physical activity leading to obesity is the important factor.[5,6]

The Women's Health Initiative demonstrated 8 more invasive breast cancers per 10,000 women in those patients that received postmenopausal hormone therapy

Table 3
Breast cancer 5-year survival rates by stage and race—NCI SEER registry years 2002 to 2008

	5-y Survival Rate by Stage and Race	
SEER Stage	White	Black
All stages	90.3%	77.7%
Localized	99.2%	92.7%
Regional	85.3%	72.9%
Distant	25.1%	15.4%
Unstaged	49.7%	44.4%

with estrogen and progestin versus women who received placebo (38/10,000 vs 30/10,000). There was no increased risk of breast cancer in women who received estrogen only. Fewer Black Americans take postmenopausal hormone replacement and, in addition, because Blacks have high hysterectomy rates, estrogen alone may be more commonly prescribed than combination therapy (estrogen plus progestin), conferring a lower breast cancer risk.[7] It is possible that some of the increased prevalence of good prognosis estrogen receptor–positive breast cancer in postmenopausal White women is due to the tendency of White women to take postmenopausal hormones.[8]

It should also be noted that breast density differs by race, but not in a pattern that explains racial differences in breast cancer risk.[9]

Several genetic factors have been identified that lead to an inherited predisposition to breast cancer.[10] Inheriting a germline mutation of BRCA1 or BRCA2 can confer an increased lifetime risk of developing breast cancer. Estimates range from 50% to 85% lifetime risk for certain mutations. More than thirteen hundred BRCA mutations have been described. Black Americans with breast cancer seem to have a different spectrum of mutations compared with those seen in Caucasians. Less than 10% of breast cancers in Black and White women are due to inherited germline mutations of BRCA1 or BRCA2.[3]

Studies of germline mutations of p53 seem to be relatively equal among the races. It thus seems that inherited mutations are not the reason for the racial disparity in breast cancer. There seems to be some racial differences in the prevalence of somatic mutations of p53. The significance of this finding is unknown.[10] The cause is likely some as yet undefined gene-environmental interaction.

Women with certain BRCA1 mutations develop cancer in their mid 30s and 40s. Their cancers tend to be high grade and triple negative, similar to cancers common in young Black women who do not have a BRCA1 mutation. There is active investigation as to whether methylation of the BRCA1 gene could inactivate it and cause these tumors in Black women.[10]

PROGNOSTIC INDICES

Even when comparing Blacks and Whites with localized disease at diagnosis, a higher proportion of Blacks are diagnosed with higher grade disease and disease with worse prognostic indices.[11] With the discovery of the her2/neu receptor and widespread use of the receptor assay, several papers started referring to a group of cancers as triple negative.[12,13] What this means is that the tumor does not express the estrogen receptor and the progesterone receptor and does not overexpress the her2/neu receptor. The first studies to show a higher proportion of Black triple-negative disease were published in the late 1990s.[10] Further analysis showed that the racial disparity in triple-negative disease is driven by a difference in estrogen receptor (ER) status. A higher proportion of White patients with breast cancer has ER-positive disease. The prevalence of cancers that express the progesterone receptor and overexpress her2/neu is the same among Black and White patients with breast cancer.

The initial studies showed that approximately 30% of Black patients with breast cancer present with triple-negative disease compared with about 20% of Whites. The higher prevalence of triple-negative disease is a concern because women with triple-negative tumors do not benefit from some of the most useful anti-breast-cancer drugs. These anti-breast-cancer drugs include hormonal therapy with the selective estrogen receptor modulators, such as tamoxifen, nor the aromatase inhibitors and the inhibitors of her2/neu, such as traztuzamab.

Today several breast cancer subtypes are recognized and have better defined prevalence in the population; these include the following:

- Basal-like (ER−, progesterone receptor negative [PR]−, human epidermal growth factor receptor-2 negative [HER2−], cytokeratin 5/6 positive, and/or HER1+),
- HER2+/ER−,
- Luminal A (ER+ and/or PR+, HER2−),
- Luminal B (ER+ and/or PR+, HER2+), and luminal B (ER+ and/or PR+, HER2+)[13]

Carey and colleagues[14] studied a large population-based cohort of patients with breast cancer. The basal-like breast cancer subtype was more prevalent among premenopausal AA women (39%) compared with postmenopausal AA women (14%) and non-AA women (16%) of any age (*P*<.001). The better prognosis, luminal A subtype was less prevalent (36% premenopausal Black vs 59% postmenopausal Black and 54% of non-Black of any age).

RACIAL DIFFERENCES IN CANCER TREATMENT

Numerous surveys of treatment patterns show that Black Americans are less likely to receive adequate care compared with White Americans.[15–17] The 2010 Centers for Disease Control and Prevention National Health Interview Survey shows that 73% of Black and White Americans aged 50 to 74 say that they had a screening mammogram within the previous 2 years (**Table 4**). There are no data to show that there is a racial difference in ability to read a mammogram. There are data to show that it is more difficult to interpret a mammogram in younger women versus older women regardless of race.[18]

Data from an equal access health care systems suggest that the provision of adequate care can close the Black-White disparity. Wojcik and colleagues[19] studied women with access to Department of Defense Hospitals. These women were wives of military retirees or military retirees themselves. In their study 24.8% of Blacks had died within 5 years of diagnosis compared with 18.1% of Whites. In the US SEER data at the time, 34.2% of Black women died within 5 years compared with 18.4% of Whites. This study suggests that socioeconomic variables play a role in the disparity between Black and White women and access to care and use of care can reduce a substantial part of the Black/White disparity. Indeed this Black population experienced a two-thirds reduction in Black-White disparity as measured in 5-year mortality statistics. Compared with Black Americans as a whole, the Black military retirees have more

Table 4	
Proportion of women aged 50 to 74 who had a mammogram in past 2 years by race/ethnicity	
All races	72.7%
White	72.8%
Black	73.2%
Asian/Pacific	64.1%
American Indian/Alaskan Native	69.4%
Hispanic	69.7%

Data from The National Health Interview Survey, Centers for Disease Control and Prevention (CDC). Cancer Screening—United States, 2010. MMWR Morb Mortal Wkly Rep 2012;61(3):41–5.

access to health care, including preventive care, and are more likely to have the education and resources to use that care. A small but significant proportion of Black patients with breast cancer refuse medical care.[17]

EQUAL TREATMENT YIELDS EQUAL OUTCOME AMONG EQUAL PATIENTS

There is good evidence that an aggressive tumor is not an inherently more aggressive disease in Black women compared with Whites. Indeed, a rule of thumb in the study of breast cancer treatment outcomes is equal treatment yields equal outcome among equal patients.[20–23] Race is not a factor in outcomes among women with the same stage and same molecular prognostic markers receiving the same treatment.

Although race need not be a factor, unfortunately, race often is a factor in outcomes. Several population-based studies have assessed the quality of care received by Black and White women.[17,24] These studies consistently show that women experience longer treatment delays after diagnosis, regardless of disease stage at diagnosis. In the study of Lund and colleagues,[17] Black women were 4 to 5 times more likely to experience delays in treatment greater than 60 days after diagnosis. Among women with localized potentially curable disease, Black women were less likely to undergo cancer-directed surgery within the first year of diagnosis compared with White women (7.5% vs 1.5%). In the same study, 39% of Blacks receiving breast-conserving surgery did not receive radiation treatment, which is generally the standard of care. Twenty-eight percent of eligible Whites did not receive radiation treatment. Black women with ER-positive disease are also less likely to receive hormonal therapy.

There is some evidence that chemotherapy doses are more often lower than recommended in Blacks compared with Whites,[25] which may be related to racial differences in the prevalence of obesity.[4]

IS RACE THE APPROPRIATE POPULATION CATEGORY?

Although it is clear that the Black population has several disparities when compared with Whites, race is an imperfect categorization. Anthropologists reject it as a scientific construct. It is not based on science (taxonomy or anthropology); it is based on societal politics and should be considered a sociopolitical categorization.[26]

Race is a construct developed about 350 years ago. The original racial categories were Negroid, Caucasoid, and Mongoloid. These categories have changed over time. Approximately 2 years before every US census, the US Office of Management and Budget defines the racial classification for US government purposes. US data are currently collected in 4 racial and one ethnic group, listed in **Table 1**. Beginning in 2000, a person can identify as more than one race but medical data are still collected in one race; this is presumably the dominant race.[26]

Other ways of categorizing populations are less political and possibly more scientific, because they better correlate with factors that more clearly influence risk of disease. These other ways of categorizing include area of geographic origin, ethnicity, and socioeconomic status.

Area of Geographic Origin

Area of geographic origin is more scientific than race. It more naturally allows for acceptance of an individual having parents and grandparents from several areas of the world.

Sickle cell disease is an example of a genetic disease that is found among people of a specific area of geographic origin. This area included sub-Saharan Africa, North Africa, the Middle East, and southern Spain, Italy, and Greece. There is a lower prevalence but a prevalence nonetheless among southern Europeans. It is not a disease of a specific race but of a specific contiguous area of geographic origin.

There are reports of women in Nigeria, Ghana, and other African countries having high rates of breast cancer at early age and more aggressive pathologic conditions. These patterns have been noted in American women of African heritage. Most Black Americans have some African, European, and Native American lineage.[27] This area of geographic origin is an active area of study.

Ethnicity

Ethnicity relates to cultural habits.[28] It can be correlated with diet, birthing, breastfeeding, and other habits. Even cigarette smoking habits vary by ethnicity. Ethnicity can often be related to area of geographic origin. Dietary differences can influence cancer risk in several ways. Studies suggest that Asians migrating to the United States have a higher incidence of several cancers compared with those who do not. Factors associated with this increase in cancer risk include changes in diet.

Socioeconomic Status

Socioeconomic status (SES) has also been shown to correlate with risk of developing disease and with outcomes from treatment of disease.[29] Indeed, in the United States, poor and lower middle class Americans tend to consume fewer fresh fruits and vegetables, and more calorie-dense processed foods, compared with the middle class. Educational differences also influence how patients consume health care.

In the United States, a higher proportion of Black Americans are poor compared with the proportion of White Americans in poverty. Race can sometimes correlate with socioeconomic status and become a confounding factor. SES is also associated with diet, lifestyle factors, physical characteristics, and even some tumor characteristics.[30]

Gordon[31] did an analysis of ER status in a cohort of primarily White American patients with breast cancer in Ohio. They found that ER-negative tumors were more common in the socioeconomically deprived. There was a similar finding in a White Scottish population.[32] An important question is, "what is it about poverty that influences breast cancer biology?" There are certainly some environmental influences that affect tumor biology. It may involve differences in diet while in childhood that can affect age of puberty. It might also involve differences in birthing habits and breast-feeding. These findings are all active leads as this is investigated.

MULTIPLE FACTORS WORKING TOGETHER

The influence of area of geographic origin, ethnicity, socioeconomic status, and even family can work together to influence risk. This influence is shown because 1.5 to 2% of women who identify themselves as of Ashkenazi Jewish decent have one of 3 specific mutations of BRCA. Intensive study of one specific mutation has shown that these women are most likely related to a woman who lived approximately six hundred years ago. Due to segregation of the population, women outside of immediate family with the mutation are distant cousins. Multiple independent events leading to the same mutation are unlikely.[33]

Recent studies suggest that risk factors for the better prognosis luminal A breast cancer were the typical risk factors for breast cancer, including low parity and older age at first full-term pregnancy. On the other hand, poorer prognosis basal-like breast cancer was associated with increased parity and younger age at first term full-term pregnancy. Longer duration breast-feeding, increasing number of children breast-fed, and increasing number of months breast-feeding per child were each associated with reduced risk of basal-like breast cancer but not a reduced risk of luminal A. Not breast-feeding and taking medications to suppress lactation were associated with increased risk of basal-like breast cancer in both premenopausal and postmenopausal women.[34] In the United States, compared with White women, a smaller proportion of Black women breast-feed. Among those who do, they are more likely to stop breast-feeding early compared with White and Hispanic Americans. Breast-feeding patterns are influenced by culture and socioeconomics.[35]

THE IMPORTANCE OF RACE IN US DATA COLLECTION

Although race is not a biologic categorization, race does matter. There has been a growing Black-White disparity in mortality after a period of relative equivalence (see **Fig. 2**). This disparity appeared after much was learned about how to screen for, detect, and treat breast cancer. A substantial literature shows that Black Americans with breast cancer are less likely to receive optimal care compared with White Americans.[16] This finding is a logistical issue. It is a very fixable reason and can resolve most of the Black-White disparity in the United States. It is most upsetting that it is still a substantial problem more than 2 decades after it was first discussed.

There are also racial differences in pathology and tumor biology causing some disparities. The reasons for the differences are not entirely known and are likely multifactorial. It can involve differences in environment in the broadest sense of the word. Differences in dietary habits, breast-feeding, obesity, and other things likely account for some of the population differences in outcome. Some familial inheritance cannot be excluded. This is an area of research that should continue, but the complexity of race must be appreciated, and the fact that area of geographic origin, ethnicity, and socioeconomic status are confounding factors, no one should assume that race is a biologic category.

REFERENCES

1. SEER Cancer Statistics Review, 1975-2009 (Vintage 2009 Populations), National Cancer Institute. Available at: http://seer.cancer.gov/csr/1975_2009_pops09/.
2. Welch HG, Schwartz LM, Woloshin S. Are increasing 5-year survival rates evidence of success against cancer? JAMA 2000;283:2975–8.
3. American Cancer Society. Breast cancer facts and figures 2011–2012. Atlanta (GA): American Cancer Society, Inc; 2012.
4. Freedman DS. Obesity - United States, 1988–2008. MMWR Surveill Summ 2011; 60(Suppl):73–7.
5. White KK, Park SY, Kolonel LN, et al. Body size and breast cancer risk: the Multiethnic Cohort. Int J Cancer 2012;131:E705–16.
6. Park SY, Kolonel LN, Henderson BE, et al. Dietary fat and breast cancer in postmenopausal women according to ethnicity and hormone receptor status: the Multiethnic Cohort Study. Cancer Prev Res (Phila) 2012;5:216–28.
7. Schairer C, Lubin J, Troisi R, et al. Menopausal estrogen and estrogen-progestin replacement therapy and breast cancer risk. JAMA 2000;283:485–91.
8. Pfeiffer RM, Mitani A, Matsuno RK, et al. Racial differences in breast cancer trends in the United States (2000–2004). J Natl Cancer Inst 2008;100:751–2.
9. Taplin SH, Rutter CM, Finder C, et al. Screening mammography: clinical image quality and the risk of interval breast cancer. AJR Am J Roentgenol 2002;178: 797–803.

10. Ademuyiwa FO, Olopade OI. Racial differences in genetic factors associated with breast cancer. Cancer Metastasis Rev 2003;22:47–53.
11. Eley JW, Hill HA, Chen VW, et al. Racial differences in survival from breast cancer. Results of the National Cancer Institute Black/White Cancer Survival Study. JAMA 1994;272:947–54.
12. Lund MJ, Trivers KF, Porter PL, et al. Race and triple negative threats to breast cancer survival: a population-based study in Atlanta, GA. Breast Cancer Res Treat 2009;113:357–70.
13. Rakha EA, Ellis IO. Triple-negative/basal-like breast cancer: review. Pathology 2009;41:40–7.
14. Carey LA, Perou CM, Livasy CA, et al. Race, breast cancer subtypes, and survival in the Carolina Breast Cancer Study. JAMA 2006;295:2492–502.
15. Rizzo M, Lund MJ, Mosunjac M, et al. Characteristics and treatment modalities for African American women diagnosed with stage III breast cancer. Cancer 2009; 115:3009–15.
16. Shavers VL, Brown ML. Racial and ethnic disparities in the receipt of cancer treatment. J Natl Cancer Inst 2002;94:334–57.
17. Lund MJ, Brawley OP, Ward KC, et al. Parity and disparity in first course treatment of invasive breast cancer. Breast Cancer Res Treat 2008;109:545–57.
18. Centers for Disease Control and Prevention (CDC). Cancer screening - United States, 2010. MMWR Morb Mortal Wkly Rep 2012;61:41–5.
19. Optenberg SA, Thompson IM, Friedrichs P, et al. Race, treatment, and long-term survival from prostate cancer in an equal-access medical care delivery system. JAMA 1995;274:1599–605.
20. Yood MU, Johnson CC, Blount A, et al. Race and differences in breast cancer survival in a managed care population. J Natl Cancer Inst 1999;91:1487–91.
21. Dignam JJ, Redmond CK, Fisher B, et al. Prognosis among African-American women and white women with lymph node negative breast carcinoma: findings from two randomized clinical trials of the National Surgical Adjuvant Breast and Bowel Project (NSABP). Cancer 1997;80:80–90.
22. Heimann R, Ferguson D, Powers C, et al. Race and clinical outcome in breast cancer in a series with long-term follow-up evaluation. J Clin Oncol 1997;15: 2329–37.
23. Franzini L, Williams AF, Franklin J, et al. Effects of race and socioeconomic status on survival of 1,332 black, Hispanic, and white women with breast cancer. Ann Surg Oncol 1997;4:111–8.
24. Coates RJ, Clark WS, Eley JW, et al. Race, nutritional status, and survival from breast cancer. J Natl Cancer Inst 1990;82:1684–92.
25. Griggs JJ, Culakova E, Sorbero ME, et al. Effect of patient socioeconomic status and body mass index on the quality of breast cancer adjuvant chemotherapy. J Clin Oncol 2007;25:277–84.
26. Brawley OW. Introduction: cancer and health disparities. Cancer Metastasis Rev 2003;22:7–9.
27. Pang J, Toy KA, Griffith KA, et al. Invasive breast carcinomas in Ghana: high frequency of high grade, basal-like histology and high EZH2 expression. Breast Cancer Res Treat 2012;135:59–66.
28. Brawley OW. Population categorization and cancer statistics. Cancer Metastasis Rev 2003;22:11–9.
29. Ward E, Halpern M, Schrag N, et al. Association of insurance with cancer care utilization and outcomes. CA Cancer J Clin 2008;58:9–31.

30. Gordon NH. Socioeconomic factors and breast cancer in black and white Americans. Cancer Metastasis Rev 2003;22:55–65.
31. Gordon NH. Association of education and income with estrogen receptor status in primary breast cancer. Am J Epidemiol 1995;142:796–803.
32. Thomson CS, Hole DJ, Twelves CJ, et al. Prognostic factors in women with breast cancer: distribution by socioeconomic status and effect on differences in survival. J Epidemiol Community Health 2001;55:308–15.
33. Berman DB, Wagner-Costalas J, Schultz DC, et al. Two distinct origins of a common BRCA1 mutation in breast-ovarian cancer families: a genetic study of 15 185delAG-mutation kindreds. Am J Hum Genet 1996;58:1166–76.
34. Millikan RC, Newman B, Tse CK, et al. Epidemiology of basal-like breast cancer. Breast Cancer Res Treat 2008;109:123–39.
35. Centers for Disease Control and Prevention (CDC). Racial and ethnic differences in breastfeeding initiation and duration, by state - National Immunization Survey, United States, 2004–2008. MMWR Morb Mortal Wkly Rep 2010;59:327–34.

Breast Cancer Risk Assessment, Prevention, and the Future

Victoria L. Green, MD, JD, MBA

KEYWORDS

- Breast cancer risk assessment • Risk models • Chemoprevention
- Preventive therapy • Nipple aspirate fluid
- Random periareolar fine-needle aspiration

KEY POINTS

- Risk assessment is recommended by the National Comprehensive Cancer Network and the United States Preventive Services Task Force for all women considering prevention of breast cancer.
- In addition to estimating a woman's future risk of breast cancer, risk-assessment models may be used to determine eligibility for clinical trials, chemoprevention, genetic testing and magnetic resonance imaging (MRI) screening.
- Breast cancer risk-assessment models largely dependent on family history, such as the Claus, BRCA Pro, BOADICEA, and Tyrer-Cuzick models, are recommended for determining those that may derive benefit from annual MRI screening.
- The combined results from the tamoxifen prevention trials shows greater than 30% reduction in the incidence of breast cancer in a high risk cohort. Overall, estrogen receptor–positive breast cancers were decreased by 48%, and this reduction benefit persisted for 10 years.
- Tamoxifen is approved by the Food and Drug Administration for breast cancer risk reduction in pre- and postmenopausal women. Raloxifene is approved for risk reduction in postmenopausal women.

INTRODUCTION

Nearly 1 in 8 women will develop breast cancer, making its diagnosis a particularly common but dreaded adversary. Breast cancer remains the leading cause of cancer in women. In the United States, more than 230,000 women will be diagnosed with breast cancer and nearly 40,000 will die from their disease. In addition, important disparities exist in that although incidence rates of breast cancer are higher in non-Hispanic white women, African American women have a higher incidence rate before

Disclosures: The author has nothing to disclose.
Department of Obstetrics and Gynecology, Gynecology Breast Clinic, Avon Comprehensive Breast Center, Winship Cancer Institute, Emory University at Grady Memorial Hospital, 69 Jesse Hill Jr Drive, Atlanta, GA 30303, USA
E-mail address: vgree01@emory.edu

Obstet Gynecol Clin N Am 40 (2013) 525–549
http://dx.doi.org/10.1016/j.ogc.2013.05.003 obgyn.theclinics.com

40 years of age and are more likely to die from breast cancer at every age.[1] Worldwide the statistics are even more alarming, with approximately 1.4 million cases and 458,000 deaths.[2] Mammographic screening has dramatically altered the landscape of the detection of breast cancer, leading to notable shifts in the diagnosis at earlier stages. However, a new paradigm is espoused, complementing the objective of early detection and treatment of breast cancer with the addition of a focus on predicting those who will develop breast cancer and offering options to prevent disease development.[3] Prevention, of course, would be a preferable alternative to treatment of established disease, particularly if those women most likely to develop breast cancer or benefit from a prevention intervention could be readily identified.

Besides the high mortality and significant morbidity of this disease, breast cancer is responsible for an extraordinarily profound emotional toll and huge personal and societal economic burden, thus highlighting the momentous public health concerns of this disease process. Advances in technology, genomics, and pharmacotherapy have made reducing the incidence and burden of breast cancer an achievable medical objective. Recent studies indicate that the incidence of breast cancer may be substantially reduced in high-risk cohorts through chemoprevention with tamoxifen or raloxifene, prophylactic oophorectomy, and prophylactic mastectomy.[4–6] However, although available strategies are clinically effective at various levels, they are often hampered by considerable side effects. Accordingly, discovering new strategies to improve the identification of women who are at high risk and thus likely to gain the most benefit from risk-reducing interventions is of critical importance.

RISK ASSESSMENT OF BREAST CANCER
Risk-Assessment Models

Attempting to gauge a woman's risk for the development of breast cancer was largely speculative for many years. A simple inventory of risk factors fails to identify a majority of women, as 70% of women with breast cancer have no identifiable risk factors other than age and gender.[7,8] Moreover, risk factors may vary by race. Studies have shown that later age at first birth and higher parity were associated with higher risk of breast cancer among African American women younger than 45 years, in comparison with the lower risk of breast cancer noted among Caucasian women in similar demographics.[9] Over the past several decades a variety of statistical models have been designed to either estimate a woman's risk of developing breast cancer or an estimation of the likelihood of harboring a heritable genetic mutation such as the BRCA gene (the significance of which is discussed in detail in the article by Meaney-Delman and Bellcross elsewhere in this issue). Model elucidation has launched an era of objective quantitative risk estimation. The goal of accurate individualized risk assessment is to have the ability to assess a particular woman's individual risk and then to appropriately tailor preventive strategies to those that will have maximal benefit with least harm. Risk assessment involves the use of statistical models and analysis of the family history to determine whether a family history is suggestive of sporadic, familial, or hereditary cancer, thus to offer the patient an individualized program of risk reduction. Risk assessment is recommended by the National Comprehensive Cancer Network (NCCN) and the United States Preventive Services Task Force (USPSTF) for all women considering prevention of breast cancer.[10] However, distilling the intricate literature can be a complex and challenging undertaking in advancing the proper clinical use of the models and preventive therapy. Important differences exist between the models, including risk factors used in analysis, United States versus European rates of breast cancer used as baseline calibrations, consideration of invasive breast cancer and ductal carcinoma in situ (DCIS) versus invasive cancers only in prediction estimation, incorporation or exclusion of lobular carcinoma in situ (LCIS), incorporation of competing mortality rates from non–breast cancer causes versus breast cancer mortality solely, and validation in the general population versus that in the high-risk population alone. Each difference possibly modifies the predicted absolute risk of breast cancer, especially over long prediction intervals. These distinctions can be critical in deciding which model to use in specific family scenarios and in interpreting the studies that assess the validity of the model.[11] In addition to their differences, the models have important limitations. Most models are based on differing combinations of traditional risk factors, although studies have shown that a majority of women with breast cancer do not have a known risk factor.[12] In addition, the risk factor may portend divergent risks for different ethnic groups.[13] Moreover, many well-established risk factors are not typically included in models. For instance, mammographic breast density is only incorporated in an adaptation of the Gail model and in the Tice model.

The Gail model is the most well-known and widely used of the risk assessment models. This model estimates a woman's risk for development of breast cancer at 5 years and the lifetime risk. The Gail model is a multivariable statistical model which is also used to determine eligibility for most chemoprevention trials, shifting its primary focus from that of risk estimation of breast cancer. A threshold of greater than 1.67% has been chosen as the level for high-risk status. In generating an estimate of risk of breast cancer the model incorporates the patient's race, age, age at menarche, age at first live birth, number of first-degree relatives with breast cancer, number of breast biopsies, and history of atypical hyperplasia. It has been shown to accurately estimate the proportion of women who will develop breast cancer when used in population studies; however, it performs poorly at discriminating between individual women who will and will not develop breast cancer.[14–16] It is limited by its inability to incorporate several important risk factors, including the age of diagnosis of disease, a family history of ovarian cancer, a family history other than a first-degree relative, Ashkenazi Jewish ancestry, a history suggestive of germline mutation, or individuals younger than 35 years. Moreover, this model may underestimate risk for younger women, carriers of BRCA mutation, and those with LCIS, DCIS, or a prior history of breast cancer. Since its initial design in 1989,[17] the Gail model has been modified to include (1) incidence rates of breast cancer in African American women, (2) incidence rates of only invasive cancer as opposed to both invasive and in situ cancers as in the initial model, and (3) age-specific incidence rates from the Surveillance, Epidemiology, and End Results (SEER) database. The original model used data from the Breast Cancer Detection and Demonstration Project (BCDDP). The Gail model has been validated in both the general population and women at high risk excluding those with LCIS, contrary to other risk-assessment models.[18] As the Gail model does not focus on family history (6 of the 7 incorporated risk factors are nonfamilial), it is generally not recommended for determining eligibility of MRI assessment in high-risk women.[19]

Because of the limitations of the Gail model, particularly for women whose predominant risk factor is a family history of breast cancer, alternative risk-assessment models such as the Claus model[20] may be a better predictor of the risk of breast cancer. By comparison, the Claus model uses genetic modeling (based on the assumption of a single autosomal dominant gene for breast cancer) to tabulate risk of breast cancer based on the age at diagnosis and number of first-degree and second-degree relatives diagnosed with breast cancer. Thus the Claus model incorporates more detailed information on family history but excludes the nonfamilial risk factors represented in the Gail model. Both models underestimate the risk of breast cancer in women who are known or suspected carriers of breast cancer susceptibility genes. In contrast to the

Gail model, the Claus model predicts the risk of both invasive and noninvasive breast cancer using data from the Cancer and Steroid Hormone Study. It allows assessment of both the maternal and paternal lineage, inclusion of second-degree relatives, and age at diagnosis of disease.[21] This model is limited, however, by lack of inclusion of hormonal and reproductive factors, incidence rates reflecting only North American risk of breast cancer, and lack of reproducibility between computerized versions and published tables. As they are largely dependent on family history, the Claus, BRCA Pro, Breast and Ovarian Analysis of Disease Incidence and Carrier Estimation Algorithm (BOADICEA), and Tyrer-Cuzick models are recommended for use in risk-reduction counseling and for determining those who may derive benefit from annual MRI screening.[22,23]

Between 9000 and 18,000 new diagnoses of breast carcinoma each year in the United States are associated with a genetically defined predisposition. BRCA 1 and BRCA 2 are highly penetrant tumor-suppressor genes accounting for 60% of inherited breast carcinomas, which portend a 36% to 85% lifetime risk for development of breast cancer and a 16% to 60% lifetime chance of developing ovarian cancer.[24–28] Gene mutations may be responsible for 5% to 10% of cases of breast cancer, and are present in less than 1% of the general population.[29] As genetic testing is expensive (US$3200–$3500) and is not recommenced in women who have a low risk of harboring a mutation,[30,31] mathematical models that predict mutation-carrier probabilities and cancer risks are used to define which individuals to test. In an attempt to improve the individual discriminatory accuracy of the Gail model, other models incorporate broader classification of risk factors and attempt to address the genetic determinants of risk. The Graham-Colditz[32,33] and Tyrer-Cuzick[34] or International Breast Cancer Intervention Study (IBIS) models use Gail model variables but add alcohol intake, age at menopause, genetic mutation status, use of hormones, extended family history of breast or ovarian cancer, age of onset, laterality of breast cancer in affected relatives, height, and body mass index. Thus the Tyrer-Cuzick model has the benefits of the Gail, BRCA Pro, and Claus models in incorporating endocrine, familial, and personal risk factors as well as allowing for the presence of multiple genes of differing penetrance. Studies have shown that the Tyrer-Cuzick model may have discriminatory value superior to that of the Gail model for women with a single affected relative.[34] However, studies have shown both overestimation and underestimation in specific populations,[33] with limited information regarding improved discriminatory accuracy in comparison with other models.[34] As each model incorporates substantially different risk factors, these models may result in substantially different estimates of risk for breast cancer.

As distinguished from estimating the probability of future breast cancer, the BOADICEA[35] and BRCA Pro[26,36] models predict the likelihood of possessing a BRCA 1 or BRCA 2 mutation. Tyrer-Cuzick predicts risk of breast cancer and the likelihood of a genetic mutation.[34] BRCA Pro is a computer-based Bayesian probability statistical model that incorporates a personal history of breast cancer, the premenopausal or postmenopausal status of affected relatives with breast or ovarian cancer, family history of male breast cancer, and Ashkenazi Jewish ancestry. Of interest, although a threshold above 10% is often used to recommend genetic testing, a significant number of mutation carriers have been found below this probability threshold, prompting questions regarding the precision of the 10% threshold. Many counselors advocate flexibility and individualization in assessing the need for testing when incorporating these factors. Although initial policy statements suggested testing for those with a probability greater than 10%, current recommendations are less stringent.[31] Moreover, similar considerations may alter application of the Gail-model risk (>1.67) in initiation of preventive interventions such as tamoxifen while balancing the adverse risks of stroke, pulmonary emboli, and endometrial cancer based on patient age. The Pedigree Assessment Tool (PAT)[37] is a method to identify patients appropriate for genetic referral by health care providers who do not specialize in cancer genetics. Although intended to be used in conjunction with existing BRCA prediction models, this model performs comparably in screening women for appropriate genetic referral.[38] In addition, its simplicity and detection of patients with non-BRCA hereditary breast cancer syndromes suggest it may be better suited for screening of breast cancer risk.

One comparison study[39] showed improved performance of BOADICEA in predicting numbers of mutations, in comparison with underestimation of mutation probability with IBIS and BRCA Pro. However, the discriminatory accuracy, measured as the area under the receiver-operating characteristic curve, was similar (0.77, 0.76, and 0.74, respectively) for each model. Additional models reviewed included Myriad II and the Manchester model, which also had similar discriminatory accuracy (0.75 and 0.72) for prediction of mutation status.[11] Investigators report deficiencies in model validation for the prediction of reliable risk estimates. Other less commonly used mutation probability models include Manchester, Penn II, Myriad II, and FHAT.

A common feature of all the models proposed to date is the lack of data measuring the distinctive individual biological information/characteristics that is unique, exclusive, and idiosyncratic to the current state of the particular women at the time of risk assessment. To improve the short-term predictive accuracy of epidemiologic models, increasing attention is being given to adding data from biological measurements (risk biomarkers) to improve the prediction of risk for breast cancer. The ultimate goal is to achieve sufficient discriminatory accuracy to appropriately target preventive therapy options, which may include chemoprevention with tamoxifen, raloxifene, and exemestane; prophylactic mastectomy/oophorectomy; MRI; and increased surveillance. In addition, modulation of predictive risk biomarkers may be used to predict and monitor response to particular prevention interventions.

Identification and modulation of phenotypic predictive markers appears to be a promising approach to improved risk assessment of breast cancer. Biomarkers are distinctive individual characteristics, often blood and tissue parameters, which can be objectively measured and tested as indicators of normal, pathologic, or pharmacologic biological processes or responses. Proposed biomarkers that could potentially add precision to risk estimation for the individual patient include serum estrogen and progesterone levels, serum insulin-like growth factor I (IGF-I) and its binding protein 3 (IGFBP-3), p53, epidermal growth factor receptor (EGFR), DNA hypermethylation of gene promoters,[40–42] bone mineral density, mammographic breast density,[43,44] and breast intraepithelial neoplasia (IEN). Each has been shown to have broader applicability than germline mutation testing (such as BRCA 1/2). However, validation of potential biomarkers has proved challenging. Mammographic breast density and breast IEN are modulatable markers, and are useful in both pre- and postmenopausal women. Breast IEN, which includes proliferative breast disease with and without atypia, atypical ductal and lobular hyperplasia, and in situ cancer, has many of the characteristics of an ideal risk biomarker and is known to be associated with an increased risk for developing breast cancer. Thus the zeal to achieve early detection of intraepithelial neoplastic changes persists unabated in the literature. Studies reveal a 4- to 5-fold increased risk of breast cancer in women with greater than 75% density on mammographic interpretation.[45] Therefore, similar to lowered low-density lipoprotein cholesterol concentrations predictive for lowered incidence of coronary heart disease among statin users, mammographic breast-density regression may be predictive of response to preventive therapy. However, mammographic breast density has been shown to add only modestly to the discriminatory accuracy of the Gail model.[46] Conversely, the Tice model incorporates breast density, which has improved model risk estimation in comparison with use of clinical factors alone.[47] Unlike the Gail model, these models have not been validated in clinical studies so counseling must stress that these figures are estimates and not absolute risks, and thus weigh the magnitude of risk for the individual patient.

Risk Assessment Using Tissue Acquisition

Although investigational at present, risk assessment for breast cancer incorporating tissue characteristics is a promising therapeutic association. The development and widespread adoption of the cervical Papanicolaou smear, based on the premise of early detection of cancerous and precancerous cellular changes, has led to a dramatic decline in mortality from cervical cancer. Similarly, it is thought that the most breast cancers (and possibly precancerous precursors) begin in the lining of the milk ducts, specifically the terminal ductal lobular units. Therefore periodic evaluation of ductal fluid theoretically should authenticate early cancerous or precancerous cell development in breast tissue, and allow the opportunity to intervene in the natural history of malignant development. The seminal work of Wrensch and Petrakis[48–50] bolstered this hypothesis, determining that women exhibiting proliferative epithelium with or without atypia in breast nipple-aspirate fluid (NAF) had a 2.4- to 2.8-fold increased risk of breast cancer compared with those who did not produce NAF (independent of traditional risk factors).[48–50] Moreover, research shows that combining NAF cytology with the Gail model has the potential to improve prediction of the incidence of breast cancer, particularly for high-risk women.[51]

Nipple aspiration is a minimally invasive procedure whereby nipple fluid is collected following 5 to 10 minutes of manual massage. Although NAF harvest requires little training, is quick, noninvasive, inexpensive, and associated with little discomfort, 15% to 50% of women do not produce NAF and of those who do produce NAF, only 27% to 84% have sufficient cells to allow morphologic characterization.[48,49,52–54] In an effort to overcome these limitations, researchers have focused on more reliable methods of obtaining epithelial cells from breast tissue and molecular (in addition to cytologic) analysis of NAF for hormone levels, proteomic patterns, and gene methylation.

Warming the breast, scrubbing the nipple to dislodge keratin plugs, and increasing the number of attempts have been advocated to improve NAF cell harvest.[55,56] In addition, specific breast pumps, similar to breast-milk pumps, have been devised with a goal of aiding NAF collection. The HALO Breast Pap Test, an automated collection apparatus approved by the Food and Drug Administration (FDA), uses latex-free sample-collection cups over an adjustable breast-suction appliance to apply gentle suction and warmth for standardized collection of NAF. The specimen is then analyzed for morphologic characteristics. In the initial study of 500 women, 38% produced NAF; however, 50% of the samples were insufficient for morphologic characterization.[57] Of those analyzed, 5 showed atypical cells. This figure translates to 1% of the study or, more simply, using HALO, 1 of 100 women tested will learn she has atypical cells and is thus at increased risk for breast cancer.[58,59] The Breast Pap Test is not touted as a diagnostic tool but is designed for use in the arena of risk assessment. Of importance is that as with all evaluations of ductal morphology, the test misses (at least) the 15% of cancers that do not arise in the ductal system (lobular). Many health insurance companies do not yet cover the cost of testing, so patients may end up about $100 out of pocket.[59]

A new generation of breast-tissue acquisition methods began with the introduction of ductal lavage (DL). DL is a minimally invasive method of collecting ductal epithelial cells for cytologic evaluation with the goal of detection of epithelial atypia to improve the precision of risk estimation of breast cancer. The efficacy of this tool is based on the premise that fluid-yielding ducts (NAF producing) are the ducts most likely to contain disease, and when these ducts are lavaged, cytologic findings may reflect the presence of disease. The hypothesis was supported by the diagnosis of cancer in 4 high-risk women undergoing DL for risk assessment without clinical or radiographic evidence of malignancy, whereby malignant cells were found in the DL effluent.[54] Although atypia identified through NAF or fine-needle aspiration (FNA) have been shown to predict an increased risk for development of breast cancer, it is unclear whether atypical cells identified through DL also indicate a similar escalation in risk. However, researchers have incorporated DL atypia to modify Gail-model risk scoring in chemoprevention trials.[60–62] In addition, investigators have delineated clinical management algorithms to address abnormal results that vary from repeat DL, recommendations for chemopreventive initiatives, ductoscopy, additional imaging, or biopsy if an abnormality is found.[62–64] However, if the algorithm is followed and no abnormality is identified, recommendations remain unclear. Moreover, in comparison with other methods of epithelial sampling, DL requires training, is relatively expensive (a catheter apparatus may cost $200–$300/per lavaged duct), and time consuming. Of note, theoretical benefits of the procedure have not been observed in critical investigation. Subsequent studies have thus not maintained the general enthusiasm for this procedure and have provided mixed reviews. Some cite appropriate feasibility of obtaining evaluable samples[65] but a lack of prognostication of DL atypia for current breast cancer[66,67]; others cite failure to yield adequate specimens sufficient for reliable cytologic diagnosis, or to support translational research activities in BRCA 1/2 women[68,69]; fair cytologic and cellular reproducibility[70–73]; and low sensitivity for detection of cancer in cancer-containing tissue.[70,74] This lack of sensitivity in a population with a high prevalence of disease may be particularly important, as it would likely present an even greater problem in a lower-prevalence population such as asymptomatic high-risk women. Proponents have previously touted the ability of repeated procedures to provide an opportunity for serial sampling and repeat biomarker analysis of the same duct over time, generally producing greater cellularity of samples than NAF and possibly greater reproducibility than random periareolar fine-needle aspiration (RPFNA). In particular, theoretically ducts can be recannulated rather than samples pooled from multiple needle passes as in the RPFNA procedure. The procedure theoretically samples an entire ductal tree rather than cells in the proximal reaches of the ductal lumen, as with NAF. Cannulation of a fluid-yielding duct is possible in 86% to 100% of women and provides specimens with greater numbers of epithelial cells, with a greater likelihood of sufficiency than NAF for cytomorphologic evaluation. Furthermore, if carefully mapped on a grid, the specific duct can be further evaluated by ductoscopy if atypical cellular material is obtained, or relavaged after chemopreventive treatments to determine cellular response to the intervention. It is this potential attribute that may set DL apart from other minimally invasive methods of obtaining specimens for risk assessment.[75–79]

DL begins with application of an anesthetic cream or injection of lidocaine subcutaneously into the nipple (nipple block).[80] Other researchers have suggested use of nitroglycerin paste to relax the nipple sphincter.[81] After gentle massage, a special suction cup attached to a syringe is placed over the nipple, and negative pressure is applied to identify fluid-producing ducts. A microcatheter is then inserted through the nipple orifice into the identified duct and is lavaged with a physiologic solution. The resultant effluent is sent for cytologic analysis.

As research continues with intraductal cannulation procedures, providers should be knowledgable of the potential for breast MRI ductal enhancement subsequent to DL, which can mimic the appearance of a carcinoma.[82]

Another method of breast epithelial sampling is RPFNA. This technique was developed to assess short-term risk of breast cancer and is grounded on the premise that widespread cellular changes within the breast might be detected by random tissue sampling. The hypothesis is supported by the multifocal, multicentric proliferative changes observed in autopsy series[83,84] and prophylactic mastectomy specimens from high-risk women.[85] Unlike DL, which assesses specific fluid-yielding ducts, RPFNA attempts to detect a field change. Initial foundational studies performed 4-quadrant FNA and noted increased cytologic evidence of proliferative breast disease in high-risk women compared with controls. RPFNA is a modification of the original technique, performing FNA at 2 sites, approximately 1 cm form the nipple areolar complex in the upper inner and upper outer quadrants of each breast.[86] Studies have supported the reproducibility of the procedure results and interinstitutional compatibility.[87] After anesthetizing the skin and subcutaneous tissues with buffered lidocaine, a 1.5-inch 21- to 23-gauge needle and a 12-mL syringe is used to perform 4 to 5 aspirations at each site. The material is pooled in a single 15-mL tube and processed for cytomorphology and biomarkers. After completion, cold packs are applied for 10 minutes and the breasts are bound firmly with soft gauze for several hours, with a tight-fitting sports bra worn for several days. Severe hematoma formation requiring surgical evacuation and/or infection requiring oral antibiotics occurred in less than 1% of aspiration visits.[88]

Finding the superior procedure for obtaining epithelial cells for risk assessment and prevention is a complicated issue without a simple answer. It depends on the skill and training of the provider, as well as the available resources for evaluation of the sample and cytology review. Overall evaluation of the breast epithelial sampling procedures reveals that NAF is less invasive than DL or RPFNA, yet DL and RPFNA yield a greater number of evaluable cells. One advantage of DL over RPFNA is the potential for investigation of specific ducts producing abnormal cellular changes via mammary ductoscopy. Using RPFNA, studies show that 94% of samples are sufficient for cytomorphologic evaluation in a high-risk cohort, compared with 60% for DL (although not in a high-risk group).[89] Furthermore, cytologic atypia on RPFNA has been shown to be associated with increased risk for future development of breast cancer; however, this has not been proved for DL atypia, although a prospective trial is currently under way to address this hypothesis. The greatest limitations of NAF are lack of NAF production and limited cellularity, which decreases the number of evaluable specimens. The greatest limitations for DL are lack of production of NAF (although non–NAF-yielding ducts may be cannulated with DL but with less success), cost, need for training, and data showing lack of reproducibility over time. The primary drawback to RPFNA is that the location of marked atypia, if observed, is unknown because samples are pooled rather than evaluated separately.

At present, the NCCN guidelines state that "the clinical utility and role of random periareolar fine-needle aspiration or ductal lavage are still being evaluated and should only be used in the context of a clinical trial."[90,79] Moreover, the National Cancer Institute states that "these techniques [nipple aspiration, ductal lavage, and fine-needle aspiration for risk assessment] are primarily research tools for obtaining epithelial cells. There is no protein or DNA biomarker from nipple aspirate fluid that is currently used in standard practice that will predict whether someone is likely to develop breast cancer"; and "there is insufficient scientific evidence to support this procedure [nipple aspiration, ductal lavage, and fine-needle aspiration for risk assessment]. Long-term studies have not been done to determine whether screening for atypical cells decreases breast cancer mortality."[91]

OncoVue is being evaluated in research as another approach to improve individualized estimation of a woman's risk for developing breast cancer and incorporating an individual's genetic assessment. This non–FDA-approved test combines 22 single-nucleotide polymorphisms (SNPs) in 19 genes with the Gail-model risk factors to arrive at an estimate of a woman's risk of breast cancer. The test is not offered direct to the consumer, as the pharmaceutical company wants to ensure clinician involvement. The OncoVue model was developed by analysis of a large case-control study genotyped for 117 common, functional SNPs in candidate genes likely to influence breast carcinogenesis. These SNPs are known to be involved in various biological pathways such as steroid hormone metabolism, DNA repair (including a BRCA1 interacting protein), cell-cycle control, apoptosis, proliferation, growth control, and detoxification. By using multivariate logistic regression analysis, the 22 candidate SNPs were identified. In initial studies OncoVue demonstrated a 2.4-fold statistically significant improvement over the Gail model by correctly placing more cases and fewer controls at elevated risk, and a 51% improvement over the Gail model in assigning elevated risk to cases.[92] OncoVue testing is performed by collecting an oral rinse and isolating DNA from buccal smears. The specimen is then analyzed with the proprietary gene SNP combination and the predictive risk analysis is sent to the patient's physician. Nevertheless, these results must be calibrated to national incidence data and validated in an independent study population before standard use in clinical practice can become possible.

Ultimately, the "true" value of any risk-prevention effort for the patient depends on the individual patient's stance regarding risk prevention. If the patient does not desire to participate in a special screening program or use preventive options, the utility of information garnered from risk assessment or genetic testing may be minimal. However, the dictum that "knowledge is power" may indicate some empowerment on the part of the patient in providing the information.

CHEMOPREVENTION/PREVENTIVE THERAPY FOR BREAST CANCER

Chemoprevention of breast cancer is an emerging area of clinical oncology addressed to healthy, unaffected individuals at higher risk for breast cancer. Pharmacologic prevention of cancer is a relatively new field but represents a very promising approach to reducing the incidence and burden of cancer. Chemoprevention can be defined as the use of specific natural or synthetic chemical agents to reverse, suppress, or prevent the progression of premalignant lesions to invasive carcinoma. It follows the example of other medical disciplines, such as cardiology whereby it is standard practice to treat individuals at higher risk for cardiovascular disorders before established clinical evidence of disease, which has contributed to decreased mortality. Adopting a similar strategy for the prevention of cancer is made possible by the expanding development of molecular drugs, which provides tools for an effective and safe molecular-targeted intervention. Development of breast cancer is a multistep, multipath, and multifocal process of genetic and epigenetic alternations leading to a series of steps from the initial status of genomic instability to the final development of cancer. The goal is now a biologically plausible concept in cancer prevention and control: to use preventive agents to interrupt the chain of molecular events in the pathogenesis of cancer before the onset of clinical disease.

The importance of prevention is clearly reflected in breast cancer statistics whereby worldwide nearly 500,000 women die yearly from breast cancer. In developing countries, where the population structure is generally younger, statistics reveal that 68,000 women younger than 40 years will die from breast cancer yearly, unlike in the Unites States where most breast cancers occur after the age of 50. Moreover, although mortality rates have declined in both the United States and the United Kingdom, rates are increasing in Singapore, Japan, and Korea, and the incidence rate has tripled over the past decade. Even within the United States, not everyone has benefited equally from the decreased mortality rate. African American women have nearly a 41% greater risk of dying from breast cancer than Caucasian women, and a nearly 50% greater risk than other minorities. In addition, efforts to find clinically applicable germline genetic variations have thus far been less revealing. Studies have yielded a few high-risk gene mutations that have extremely low prevalence (BRCA 1, BRCA 2, TP53, PTEN). These mutations are important for individual families but have a small attributable risk in the general population. Of note, approximately 2240 men will be afflicted with breast cancer and 410 will die from their disease.[1,93]

As the terminology chemoprevention evokes connotations of cancer and chemotherapy, investigators are espousing a movement toward an umbrella term of "preventive therapy," which incorporates surgical, pharmacologic, and nonpharmacologic interventions such as reducing obesity, breastfeeding, moderating alcohol intake, and increasing physical activity. These interventions have benefits in not only the general population but also those at high risk and those with germline mutations.[94] The surgical and nonpharmacologic interventions are reviewed in more detail in articles by Brawley and Meany Delman elsewhere in this issue.

At present, primary pharmacologic prevention of breast cancer rests with the selective estrogen receptor modulators (SERMs). When tamoxifen was introduced nearly 40 years ago, it revolutionized the treatment of early-stage breast cancer. At that time tamoxifen was shown to reduce the risk of recurrence in the affected breast, reduce the incidence of new primaries in the contralateral breast, and reduce mortality rates in patients with early breast cancer. In addition, a 40% higher disease-free survival rate was noted in tamoxifen-treated patients.[95] Thus tamoxifen became an obvious candidate for assessment in the prevention arena, resulting in the first prevention trial by the National Surgical Adjuvant Breast and Bowel Project (NSABP-P1 trial) or Breast Cancer Prevention Trial (BCPT). Eligible candidates for the trial were chosen based on Gail-model risk greater than 1.66%, age between 35 and 60 years, or history of LCIS. This randomized, placebo-controlled trial resulted in a highly statistically significant 49% reduction in invasive breast cancer using 20 mg tamoxifen per day in the 13,388 healthy unaffected high-risk women studied.[4] The reduction was noted solely in estrogen receptor (ER)-positive cancers after a median follow-up of 54.6 months. There was also a 45% reduction in the incidence of hip fractures but no effect on the likelihood of ischemic heart disease. An increased number of vascular events was noted, although patients with history of deep vein thrombosis (DVT) and pulmonary embolism (PE) were excluded in the initial randomization. The results were unblinded after the initial report, and participants in the placebo arm were offered tamoxifen. Subsequent analysis of the additional follow-up showed a 43% reduction in incidence of invasive breast cancer in the tamoxifen-treated group, although the unblinding may have compromised the result.[96] Ultimately, however, the results did not show an impact on survival in tamoxifen-treated patients, despite the reduction in risk of breast cancer noted.

This benefit of tamoxifen use was later confirmed by the International Breast Cancer Intervention Study (IBIS-I). This randomized, placebo-controlled study showed a 32%

reduction in all breast cancer events in 7152 high-risk women. However, the reduction was not statistically significant for invasive cancers. Eligibility criteria were similar to those of the NSABP-P1 trial.[97,98]

By contrast, the Royal Marsden Tamoxifen Prevention Trial did not initially replicate the benefits noted in the NSABP-P1 and IBIS-I trials.[99] In a smaller number of women (N = 2471), selected solely on the basis of a family history of breast cancer, there were no benefits to tamoxifen therapy after a median follow-up of 70 months. Important in this study, there was an appreciable rate of noncompliance (26%) and fewer older women (12%) compared with 31% in the NSABP-P1 trial. However, after a 13-year extended follow-up (20 years total counting the initial pilot trial) a statistically significant reduction in the incidence of ER-positive breast cancer was observed in tamoxifen-treated patients, which occurred predominantly during the posttreatment follow-up. This result indicates the long-term prevention of estrogen-dependent breast cancer by tamoxifen rather than a treatment effect of tamoxifen on estrogen-dependent disease. However, the study did not demonstrate a statistically significant advantage of tamoxifen over placebo in the prevention of invasive cancer (ER-positive and ER-negative) overall.[100]

The Italian National Trial randomized 5408 healthy hysterectomized women between the ages of 35 and 70 years to tamoxifen.[101] This study showed no effect in this group of low-risk women after a median follow-up of 81.2 months.[102] The investigators suggest that these women may well have been protected naturally by late age of menarche, early first pregnancy, or possible attendant oophorectomy (as oophorectomy may have been performed concordantly because hysterectomy was a requirement for inclusion in the study).

The combined results from the 4 tamoxifen prevention trials show a 38% reduction in the incidence of breast cancer. Overall, ER-positive breast cancers decreased by 48%, and this reduction benefit persisted for 10 years. No benefit was noted in ER-negative cancers.[103] Of note, there was no effect on all-cause mortality in the tamoxifen prevention trials, but these trials were neither designed nor statistically powered to assess mortality as an outcome or to detect this difference. Nevertheless, a reduction in the incidence of breast cancer is thought to be a noteworthy health outcome in and of itself. Thus 3 of 4 prevention trials now show a reduction in breast cancer events, although there were differences in age of eligibility as well as level of risk for selection in each of the trials. For instance, in the Royal Marsden trial the family history could have occurred in a second-degree relative rather than the significantly elevated risk noted for women with Gail-model risk greater than 1.67 as used for the NSABP-P1 and IBIS-I trials. In addition, hormone replacement therapy was excluded in NSABP-P1 but was allowed in the Italian trial. Tamoxifen has now been approved by the FDA since 1998 for breast cancer risk reduction, both invasive and noninvasive, in both pre- and postmenopausal women, with a 10-year efficacy (although only taken for 5 years, the benefit extends for at least 10 years). Because of its proven effectiveness sand well-understood toxicity profile, tamoxifen is presently deemed to be the preventive agent of choice in most high-risk women, especially in premenopausal women or those with atypical hyperplasia or LCIS, or with a history of hysterectomy. Tamoxifen is contraindicated in women with acute or prior history of DVT, PE, stroke, and transient ischemic attack.

Concomitantly, another SERM, raloxifene, was being studied in the Multiple Outcomes of Raloxifene evaluation (MORE) for prevention of osteoporosis and decreased fracture rate in 7705 postmenopausal women with a mean age of 66 years, who were entered into the trial regardless of risk of breast cancer. A 62% reduction in breast cancer was shown.[104] The trial continued as the Continuing Outcomes Relevant to Evista (CORE) trial, again showing a 58% reduction in breast cancer in comparison with placebo.[105] The RUTH (Raloxifene Use for The Heart) trial investigated reduction in cardiovascular events and the incidence of invasive breast cancer in 10,101 postmenopausal women with risk factors for coronary heart disease.[106] A 33% reduction in breast cancer overall, 44% reduction in invasive breast cancer, and a 55% reduction in ER-positive breast cancer was shown. There was no effect on ER-negative breast cancer or noninvasive breast cancer. The benefits in these studies prompted a head-to-head comparison of tamoxifen and raloxifene in the Study of Tamoxifen and Raloxifene (STAR) NSABP-P2 trial.[107] A total of 19,000 high-risk women were randomized to either 20 mg tamoxifen or 60 mg raloxifene daily. Both drugs were shown to reduce the risk of developing invasive breast cancer by about 50%; however, raloxifene was shown to have 36% fewer uterine cancers and 29% fewer blood clots than in the group assigned to tamoxifen. Thus it appears that tamoxifen and raloxifene are equally efficacious in reducing the risk of invasive breast cancer, but only tamoxifen has been shown to reduce the risk also of noninvasive cancer. The mechanism of action is not well understood. The toxicity profile is more favorable with raloxifene, although both drugs increase a woman's risk of DVT, stroke, ischemic heart disease, and PE. Only tamoxifen is associated with an increased risk of uterine cancers and cataract formation. The side effects of tamoxifen are greatest in women older than 50 years, therefore tamoxifen is often reserved for those premenopausal high-risk women with precancerous risk factors such as atypical hyperplasia or LCIS. Raloxifene may be most efficacious in the postmenopausal woman with osteoporosis for reduction of invasive breast cancer. At present, unlike tamoxifen, raloxifene has not demonstrated activity in noninvasive disease, established breast cancer, or recurrent breast cancer, or for the treatment of breast cancer.

With the SERMs generally, there are conflicting studies regarding breast cancer risk reduction, and overall no survival benefit has been shown. In addition to uterine cancer, tamoxifen is also associated with thromboembolic events, cataract formation, increased vaginal discharge/bleeding, hot flashes, leg cramps, and bladder-control problems, primarily stress urinary incontinence.[108] Information regarding the influence of tamoxifen on cognition comes from reports NSABP B14 and B20 which, although suggesting negative effects, are unable to adequately control for potential confounding factors. Thus the reported effects of tamoxifen on cognition are inconclusive at this stage. Conversely, raloxifene is more likely to be associated with increased musculoskeletal problems (joint pain, muscle stiffness), dyspareunia (vaginal dryness), and weight gain. Although tamoxifen has been used for 5 years in oncology for women with breast cancer, it is as yet unknown as to whether 5 years is the optimal therapy duration for preventive therapy in the unaffected high-risk individual, although this is currently the standard pattern of preventive use. Moreover, studies have not determined the proper age to start therapy nor the risk level suggested for initiation of therapy. Many investigators have suggested a 10-year risk of 4% to 8% for developing breast cancer to initiate preventive therapy, although this is theoretical.[109]

Similar reduction of breast cancer in tamoxifen-treated BRCA-mutation carriers has also been shown. Preliminary data in BRCA-mutation carriers affected with breast cancer showed that tamoxifen protected against contralateral breast cancer for carriers of BRCA 1 mutations (62%) and with BRCA 2 mutations (37% reduction). Overall, in women who used tamoxifen for 2 to 4 years the risk of contralateral breast cancer was reduced by 75%. Therefore, in this study tamoxifen use reduced the risk of contralateral breast cancer in women with pathogenetic mutations in either the BRCA 1 or BRCA 2 gene.[110] Other studies have shown benefit in only BRCA 2 carriers. The lack of benefit in BRCA 1 carriers is thought to be secondary to a higher likelihood of ER-negative tumors in BRCA 1 carriers.

Aromatase inhibitors reduce the biosynthesis of estrogen and in oncology, and have shown superior efficacy to tamoxifen in decreasing contralateral breast cancer events in patients with early-stage breast cancer. In general, aromatase inhibitors have over-taken tamoxifen as the treatment of choice in the postmenopausal patient with hormone-responsive breast cancer, secondary to improved efficacy over tamoxifen in reduction of recurrence of breast cancer and contralateral tumors.[111–115] Aromatase inhibitors are thus poised to make an exciting contribution in the primary prevention arena. The Mammary Prevention trial 3 (MAP 3) is a randomized, double-blind, pla-cebo-controlled, multicenter, multinational trial in which 4560 high-risk postmeno-pausal women were randomly assigned to either placebo or exemestane 25 mg daily for a median of 3 years. Investigators found a 65% relative reduction in the annual occurrence of invasive breast cancer with exemestane in comparison with placebo, and a 53% reduction in invasive plus noninvasive breast cancer. There was a 5% noncompliance rate in each group.[116] The benefit/risk ratio for use of exemestane is influenced by age, bone density, and comorbid conditions. Although exemestane is not currently FDA approved for breast cancer risk reduction, it is included as one of the choices of risk-reduction agents by the NCCN.[117]

Aromatase inhibitors are associated with an increased risk of musculoskeletal side effects in comparison with tamoxifen. The specific effects of exemestane on bone were reviewed in a subset of women from the MAP 3 trial. The study enrolled 351 healthy high-risk postmenopausal women randomized to exemestane (an aromatase inhibitor) versus placebo at 3 centers in Canada. Only 7.6% had a Gail-model risk greater than 1.67, and the average age was 61 years. A 3-fold age-related bone loss was noted on comparing baseline bone mineral density scores with those 2 years posttreatment with exemestane. During the study, women had adequate calcium and vitamin D intake. There was no increased fracture rate in comparison with pla-cebo, so the clinical significance of the finding is not clear; however, the investigators suggest women who are considering exemestane for prevention of breast cancer should have their bone health monitored during treatment, and maintain adequate cal-cium and vitamin D intake.[118] The NCCN also supports baseline evaluation of bone mineral density in postmenopausal women choosing an aromatase inhibitor for risk reduction.[119] Other adverse effects of exemestane are generally mild, with the most common being diarrhea, joint pain, and menopausal-related symptoms. Exemestane did not increase the risk of endometrial cancers, thromboembolism, cardiovascular events, or cataracts. However, joint stiffness and arthralgia were more common when compared with tamoxifen or raloxifene.[120] Thus pharmacologic preventive ther-apy may be associated with side effects that must be assessed to determine whether the benefits are greater than the risks. Final results of the IBIS-2 trial,[121] reviewing ran-domized controlled use of the aromatase inhibitor anastrazole in comparison with pla-cebo in postmenopausal high-risk women, are anxiously awaited.[122] Use of aromatase inhibitors is restricted to postmenopausal women at present, because in premeno-pausal women high levels of androstenedione compete with the aromatase inhibitor at the enzyme complex such that estrogen synthesis is not completely blocked. In addition, the initial decrease in estrogen levels causes a reflex increase in gonado-tropin levels, provoking ovarian hyperstimulation, thereby increasing aromatase in the ovary and consequently overcoming the initial aromatase blockade.

Considering current information regarding pharmacologic risk reduction (despite conflicting results and known side effects), the American Society of Clinical Oncology (ASCO) recommends discussion of pharmacologic intervention for breast cancer risk reduction in high-risk women (Gail model >1.66% or history of LCIS, atypical ductal hyperplasia) at risk for ER-positive breast cancer, as part of a shared decision-making process with "careful consideration of individually calculated risks and benefits."[123] ASCO recommendations include a gynecologic examination before initiation of pharmacologic preventive therapy and annually thereafter. Prompt evaluation of abnormal vaginal bleeding is critical, although yearly endometrial assessment is not required in the asymptomatic patient. The NCCN also recommends an ophthalmology examination if cataracts or vision problems exist, with considerations for monitoring for loss of bone mineral density if premenopausal, in addition to monthly breast self-examination, clinical breast examination every 6 months for symptoms, and annual mammography.

THE FUTURE OF CARE IN PREVENTION OF BREAST CANCER

Prevention of breast cancer is a rapidly evolving area of cancer control. Retinoids have been studied as preventive agents in clinical trials because of their established role in regulating cell growth, differentiation, and apoptosis in preclinical models.[124] Fenretinide is the most widely studied retinoid in breast cancer prevention trials, because of its selective accumulation in breast tissue and its favorable toxicologic profile. Fenretinide is a vitamin A analogue that has shown benefit in a phase III study of 3000 women aged 30 to 70 years with DCIS or early stage I breast cancer (this was not a prevention study, as patients were already diagnosed with breast cancer). Women were randomized to ingesting 200 mg per day of fenretinide in comparison with placebo, and although there was no statistically significant reduction in overall incidence of breast cancer, there was a trend toward reduction in premenopausal risk of breast cancer. Side effects included dermatologic conditions (skin or mucosal dryness, pruritus, urticaria, and dermatitis) and diminished dark-vision adaptations. Despite the encouraging preliminary results regarding breast cancer risk reduction, however, fenretinide is not approved for risk reduction in the United States. Retinoids may represent more effective and tolerable agents for the prevention of ER-negative breast cancer.[125]

There has been a wealth of supporting epidemiologic and laboratory data touting the favorable effects of soy consumption, noted mainly in the Asian population, thus making soy isoflavones a prime dietary candidate for evaluation of the prevention of breast cancer. However, rodent data suggesting a cancer-promoting effect has deterred further study and portend cautious intake of soy in survivors of breast cancer. A recent randomized phase II placebo-controlled trial of breast cancer risk reduction used RPFNA to obtain breast epithelial cells for the measurement of proliferation activity (as measured by Ki67 levels). Levels measured before and after a 6-month intervention of processed soy intake showed no favorable effects of modulation of the Ki67 biomarker. By contrast, the same agent in the same dose and schedule had produced favorable modulation of a different biomarker (MMP2) in a trial of prostate cancer, thus highlighting the potential organ specificity of preventive agents. Investigators surmise that the lack of modulation may be due to a need to mimic routine patterns of intake, which would generally occur in divided daily doses rather than the single ingested dose used in the trial. In addition, most individuals consume whole soy rather than a processed/mixed supplement. Moreover, the beneficial effects of soy anecdotally seem to be derived from exposure early in life rather than late supplementation in the diets of Western women, which currently appears to have minimal impact. Future research should therefore focus on smaller doses throughout the day, whole soy, and exposure early in life.[126] Using a different lignan (secoisolariciresinol diglycoside), researchers were able to show a beneficial effect in reduction of Ki67 in benign breast tissue of high-risk women, with lack of adverse events. This result has now prompted a randomized, placebo-controlled trial in premenopausal high-risk women.[127]

The main target of nonsteroidal anti-inflammatory drugs (NSAIDs) is the cyclooxygenase (COX)-1 and COX-2 receptors. Numerous studies have tested the cancer-preventive effects of various NSAIDs and selective COX-2 inhibitors, with some selective COX-2 inhibitors showing significant reduction in the incidence and multiplicity of rat mammary tumors. Use of celecoxib (a selective COX-2 inhibitor) in mice has been shown to reduce basal cell carcinoma lesions by 30%. Additional studies in humans have produced similar beneficial results with long-term use of other COX-2 inhibitors, other NSAIDs, and aspirin.[128] The risk of thrombotic cardiovascular events (including a slight increased risk of myocardial infarction) associated with selective COX-2 inhibitors has slowed studies using this method.[129]

It is known that 1,25-dihydroxyvitamin D has a wide range of biological actions and that the vitamin D receptor is present in most tissues and cells in the body. Therefore, it was not unexpected that multiple studies have associated vitamin D deficiency with many types of cancer. A recent study of women in Marin County, California (which has a very high incidence of breast cancer) noted a high frequency of the VDR Apa1 A2/A2 homozygous polymorphism in women designated as at elevated risk for breast cancer by the polyfactorial risk model OncoVue. Investigators surmise that the high incidence rates in this population could be modified by vitamin D supplementation.[130]

The statins are a class of cholesterol-lowering medications and are among the most commonly prescribed drugs in the United States. Statins are safe, nontoxic, and effective agents for cholesterol lowering, and appear to have anticancer effects. A diverse body of laboratory data suggests that the statins may have chemopreventive potential against cancer at various sites, including colon, lung, breast, and prostate.[131] However, limited study of statin use has yielded mixed results,[132–135] although benefit has been noted in certain epidemiologic studies for ER-negative cancers[136] as well as early-stage high-grade lesions when evaluating fluvastatin use on measurement of breast epithelial cell proliferation (measured by Ki67 reduction). Fluvastatin shows measurable biological changes by inhibiting tumor proliferation and increasing apoptotic activity in high-grade stage 0/1 breast cancer. No benefit was noted in low-grade tumors.[137]

Future research must continue to investigate pharmacologic preventive therapy that may aim at other molecular targets such as tyrosine kinases, angiogenic factors such as vascular endothelial growth factor receptor, poly(ADP-ribose)polymerase inhibitors (which have shown some benefit in BRCA-mutation carriers), and 3-hydroxy-3-methylglutaryl coenzyme A. In addition, continued evaluation of non–FDA-approved drugs is required, such as tibolone,[138] arzoxifene,[139] and lasofoxifene,[140] which have been shown to be beneficial in reducing breast cancer, as well as metformin[141,142] and bisphosphanates.[143,144] Further study of all methods is needed, particularly in ER-negative females where applicable. ER-negative breast cancer accounts for 30% of breast cancer in Caucasian women, and an even higher proportion of cancers (40%) in the African American population. Current data show that these cancers are generally not affected by SERMs. Focus must remain on reducing adverse events associated with SERMs, aromatase inhibitors, and other pharmacologic interventions for prevention. In addition, because of the large number of women needed for powered calculations in prevention studies, increased use of biomarker modulation (such as Ki67 for measurement of proliferation activity) is required to estimate the efficacy of interventions in cohorts or women with breast cancer or at high risk.[145] Further study of appropriate risk-reduction biomarkers is key.

Vaccines for Breast Cancer

Vaccines represent an attractive therapeutic strategy for the prevention of breast cancer, as theoretically they are more specific and less toxic than chemotherapy.

Innovative evolutions in tumor immunology and molecular characterization of breast cancers have advanced the possibility of in vivo therapeutics targeted at tumor-associated antigens (TAA). These TAAs then serve as the target for the immune response and as a platform for antigen delivery. Incorporation of immunoadjuvants assists in promoting an environment conducive to immune stimulation (enhancing a robust immune response to the targeted antigen). The patient's immune system will then recognize and destroy tumor cells expressing the target antigen. The associated T-cell memory response could potentially allow for sustained effect without repeated therapy and a renewed response in the event of tumor recurrence. This aspect is of notable importance, as a significant proportion of patients with breast cancer will suffer recurrence despite advances in standard treatment regimens, and ultimately will succumb to their disease.

Renewed enthusiasm in vaccine technology has been prompted by the success of sipuleucil-T, an autologous cellular vaccine, which demonstrated a 22% relative reduction in the risk of death compared with placebo when administered to patients with hormone refractory metastatic prostate cancer.[146] Conversely, early clinical trials to evaluate cancer vaccines failed to demonstrate substantial clinical efficacy, with dismally low objective response rates of less than 5%.[147] Immunotherapy treatments are not new in the field of breast disease because the HER2/neu protein is targeted by trastuzumab, a monoclonal antibody, which has made momentous strides in treatment of HER2-overexpressing disease. At present there are more than 25 National Cancer Institute active breast cancer phase I and II vaccine trials.[148]

SUMMARY

Risk assessment of breast cancer is a burgeoning science. At present, models incorporating both personal history and genetic determinants may be used to estimate a woman's risk of developing breast cancer or to determine appropriate testing for BRCA 1 or BRCA 2. However, use of breast-tissue sampling for risk assessment is evolving, and should be limited to clinical trials until further data substantiate its ability to determine women at increased risk. The obstetrician-gynecologist is in a unique position to initiate a discussion of risk assessment of breast cancer and its prevention with their patients, so it is critical that they be familiar with the evolving science of risk assessment of breast cancer, as well as the quantitative approaches and interventional and surveillance strategies. Despite the excitement regarding significant advances in breast cancer, we must have an acute awareness of the preliminary nature of much of our knowledge regarding the clinical application in these rapidly emerging fields of risk assessment, molecular genetics, and genomics of breast cancer. Thus one must assess the literature with an appreciation of the need for flexibility when applying the information to individual families. Long-term safety and quality of life will be important end points in future studies. Genomics is poised to become a major force in cancer care, and therapy guided by genetics is being embraced within established strategies for the treatment and prevention of several malignancies.

REFERENCES

1. American Cancer Society. *Cancer Facts & Figures 2013*. Atlanta (GA): American Cancer Society; 2013. Available at: http://www.cancer.org/research/cancerfacts statistics/cancerfactsfigures2013/index. Accessed August 3, 2013.
2. American Cancer Society. Global cancer facts & figures. 2nd edition. Atlanta (GA): American Cancer Society; 2011.

3. American College of Obstetricians and Gynecologists. Breast cancer prevention and treatment: what's new, what's promising. ACOG Today 2003;47(9):1.
4. Fisher B, Costantino JP, Wickerham DL, et al. Tamoxifen for prevention of breast cancer: report of the National Surgical Adjuvant Breast and Bowel Project P-1 Study. J Natl Cancer Inst 1998;90(18):1371–88.
5. Hartmann LC, Schaid DJ, Woods JE, et al. Efficacy of bilateral prophylactic mastectomy in women with a family history of breast cancer. N Engl J Med 1999;14:71–84.
6. Rebbeck TR, Levin AM, Eisen A, et al. Breast cancer risk after bilateral prophylactic oophorectomy in *BRCA1* mutation carriers. J Natl Cancer Inst 1999;91: 1475–9 (IIa, B).
7. Collaborative Group on Hormonal Factors in Breast Cancer. Familial breast cancer: collaborative reanalysis of individual data from 52 epidemiological studies including 58.209 women with breast cancer and 101,986 women without the disease. Lancet 2001;358(9291):1389–99.
8. Green VL. Breast diseases: benign and malignant. In: Rock JA, Jones HW III, editors. TeLinde's operative gynecology. 10th edition. Philadelphia: Lippincott Williams & Wilkins; 2008. p. 1163–223.
9. Palmer JR, Wise LA, Horton NJ, et al. Dual effect of parity on breast cancer risk in African-American women. J Natl Cancer Inst 2003;95:478–83.
10. U.S. Preventive Services Task Force. Chemoprevention of breast cancer: recommendations and rationale. Ann Intern Med 2002;137:56–8.
11. Gail MH, Nai PL. Comparing breast cancer risk assessment models. J Natl Cancer Inst 2010;102(10):665–8.
12. Madigan MR, Ziegler RG, Benichou J, et al. Proportion of breast cancer cases in the United States explained by well-established risk factors. J Natl Cancer Inst 1995;87(22):1681–5.
13. McCullough ML, Feigelson HS, Diver WR, et al. Risk factors for fatal breast cancer in African-American women and white woman in a large US prospective cohort. Am J Epidemiol 2005;162(8):734–42.
14. Costantino JP, Gail MH, Pee D, et al. Validation studies for models projecting the risk of invasive and total breast cancer incidence. J Natl Cancer Inst 1999;91: 1541–8.
15. Rockhill B, Spiegelman D, Byrne C, et al. Validation of the Gail et al model of breast cancer risk prediction and implications for chemoprevention. J Natl Cancer Inst 2001;93:358–66.
16. Spiegelman D, Colditz GA, Hunter D, et al. Validation of the Gail et al. model for predicting individual breast cancer risk. J Natl Cancer Inst 1994;86:600–7.
17. Gail MH, Brinton LA, Byar DP, et al. Projecting individualized probabilities of developing breast cancer for white females who are being examined annually. J Natl Cancer Inst 1989;81(24):1879–86.
18. Amir E, Freedman OC, Seruga B, et al. Assessing women at high risk of breast cancer: a review of risk assessment models. J Natl Cancer Inst 2010;102(10): 680–91.
19. NCCN clinical practice guidelines in oncology. Breast cancer risk reduction version 1.2012. BRISK 2 ref i. Available at: http://www.nccn.org/professionals/ physician_gls/pdf/breast_risk.pdf. Accessed March 17, 2013.
20. Claus EB, Schidkraut JM, Thompson QW, et al. The genetic attributable risk of breast and ovarian cancer. Cancer 1996;77:2318.
21. Claus EB, Risch N, Thompson WD. Autosomal dominant inheritance of early onset breast cancer: implications for risk prediction. Cancer 1994;73(3):643–51.

22. National Comprehensive Cancer Network Guidelines Version 1/2012. Breast cancer risk reduction. Available at: http://www.nccn.org/professionals/physician_gls/f_guidelines.asp#detection. Accessed February 9, 2013.

23. Saslow D, Boetes C, Burke W, et al. American Cancer Society guidelines for breast screening with MRI as an adjunct to mammography. CA Cancer J Clin 2007;57:75–89.

24. Antoniou A, Pharoah PD, Narod S, et al. Average risks of breast and ovarian cancer associated with BRCA 1 and BRCA 2 mutations detected incase series unselected for family history: a combined analysis of 22 studies. Am J Hum Genet 2003;72:117–23.

25. King MC, Marks JH, Mandell JB, et al. Breast and ovarian cancer risks due to inherited mutations in BRCA 1 and BRCA 2. Science 2003;302:643–6.

26. Chen S, Parmigiani G. Meta-analysis of BRCA 1 and BRCA 2 penetrance. J Clin Oncol 2007;25(11):1329–33.

27. Levy-Lahad E, Friedman E. Cancer risks among BRCA 1 and BRCA 2 mutation carriers. Br J Cancer 2007;96(1):11–5.

28. Jatoi I, Anderson WF. Management of women who have a genetic predisposition for breast cancer. Surg Clin North Am 2008;88:845–61.

29. Rebbeck TR. The contribution of inherited genotype to breast cancer. Breast Cancer Res 2002;4:85–9.

30. American Society of Clinical Oncology. Policy statement update: genetic testing for cancer susceptibility. J Clin Oncol 2003;21(12):2397–406.

31. Nelson HD, Huffman LH, Fu R, et al. Genetic risk assessment and BRCA mutation testing for breast and ovarian cancer susceptibility: systematic evidence review for the US Preventive Services Task Force. Ann Intern Med 2005;143(5):362–79.

32. Colditz GA, Rosner B. Cumulative risk of breast cancer to age 70 years according to risk factor status: data from the Nurses' Health Study. Am J Epidemiol 2000;152:950–64.

33. Rosner B, Colditz GA. Nurses' health study: log-incidence mathematical model of breast cancer incidence. J Natl Cancer Inst 1996;88:359–64.

34. Tyrer J, Duffy SW, Cuzick J. A breast cancer prediction model incorporating familial and personal risk factors. Stat Med 2004;23(7):1111–30.

35. Antoniou AC, Cunningham AP, Peto J, et al. The BOADICEA model of genetic susceptibility to breast and ovarian cancers: updates and extensions. Br J Cancer 2008;98(8):1457–66.

36. Berry DA, Parmigiani G, Sanchaez J, et al. Probability of carrying a mutation of breast-ovarian cancer gene BRCA1 based family history. J Natl Cancer Inst 1997;89(3):227–38.

37. Available at: www.mybreastrisk.com. Accessed November 5, 2009.

38. Teller P, Stanislaw C, Green VL, et al. Validation of the Pedigree Assessment Tool (PAT) in families with BRCA1 and BRCA 2 mutations. Ann Surg Oncol 2010;17(1):240–6.

39. Antoniou AC, Hardy R, Walker L, et al. Predicting the likelihood of carrying a BRCA1 or BRCA2 mutation: validation of BOADICEA, BRCAPro, IBIS, myriad and the Manchester scoring system using data from UK genetics clinics. J Med Genet 2008;45(7):425–31.

40. Fackler MJ, Malone K, Zhang Z, et al. Quantitative multiplex methylation specific PCR analysis doubles detection of tumor cells in breast ductal fluid. Clin Cancer Res 2006;12:3306–10.

41. Bean GR, Scott V, Yee L, et al. Retinoic acid receptor beta 2 promoter methylation in random periareolar fine needle aspiration. Cancer Epidemiol Biomarkers Prev 2005;14:790–8.
42. Lewis CM, Cler LR, Bu DW, et al. Promoter hypermethylation in benign breast epithelium in relation to predicted breast cancer risk. Clin Cancer Res 2005; 11:166–72.
43. Pinsky RW, Helvie MA. Mammographic breast density: effect on imaging and breast cancer risk. J Natl Compr Canc Netw 2010;8:1157–65.
44. Chiu SY, Duffy S, Yen AM, et al. Effect of baseline breast density on breast cancer incidence, stage mortality, and screening parameters: 25 year follow up of a Swedish mammographic screening. Cancer Epidemiol Biomarkers Prev 2010; 19:1219–28.
45. Kim J, Han W, Moon H, et al. Breast density change as a predictive surrogate for response to adjuvant endocrine therapy in hormone receptor positive breast cancer. Breast Cancer Res 2012;14:403.
46. Tice JA, Ziv E, Kerlikowske KM. Mammographic breast density combined with the Gail model for breast cancer risk prediction. Breast Cancer Res Treat 2004;88(Suppl 1):S11 [abstract 13].
47. Tice JA, Cummings SR, Smith-Bindman R, et al. Using clinical factors and mammographic breast density to estimate breast cancer risk: development and validation of a new predictive model. Ann Intern Med 2008;148(5):337–47.
48. Wrensch MR, Petrakis NL, King EB, et al. Breast cancer incidence in women with abnormal cytology in nipple aspirates of breast fluid. Am J Epidemiol 1992;135:130–41.
49. Wrensch MR, Petrakis NL, Miike R, et al. Breast cancer risk in women with abnormal cytology in nipple aspirates of breast fluid. J Natl Cancer Inst 2001; 93:1791–8.
50. Buehring GC, Letscher A, McGirr KM, et al. Presence of epithelial cells in nipple aspirate fluid associated with subsequent breast cancer: a 25 year prospective study. Breast Cancer Res Treat 2006;98:63–70.
51. Tice JA, Miike R, Adduci K, et al. Nipple aspirate fluid cytology and the Gail model for breast cancer risk assessment in a screening population. Cancer Epidemiol Biomarkers Prev 2005;14(2):324–8.
52. Dooley WC, Ljung BM, Veronesi U, et al. Ductal lavage for detection of cellular atypia in women at high risk for breast cancer. J Natl Cancer Inst 2001;93:1624–32.
53. Sharma P, Klemp JR, Simonsen M, et al. Failure of high risk women to produce nipple aspirate fluid does not exclude detection of cytologic atypia in random periareolar fine needle aspiration specimens. Breast Cancer Res Treat 2004; 87:59–64.
54. Francescatti DS, Kluskens L, Shah L. Ductal lavage using medically aseptic technique in a woman at high risk for breast cancer. Clin Breast Cancer 2004; 5:299–302.
55. King EB, Chew KL, Hom JD, et al. Multiple sampling for increasing the diagnostic sensitivity of nipple aspirate fluid for atypical cytology. Acta Cytol 2004; 48:813–7.
56. Sartorius OW, Smith HS, Morris P, et al. Cytologic evaluation of breast fluid in the detection of breast disease. J Natl Cancer Inst 1977;59:1073–80.
57. Proctor KA, Rowe LR, Bentz JS. Cytologic features of nipple aspirate fluid using an automated non-invasive collection device: a prospective observational study. BMC Womens Health 2005;5:10.

58. Hamel PJ. Risk detection: how does halo measure up? Available at: www. healthcentral.com/breast-cancer/c/78/64158/detection-halo/pf/. Accessed March 23, 2009.
59. Available at: http://breastcancer.about.com/od/risk/tp/haol_breast_pap_exam. htm. Accessed October 5, 2009.
60. West JG, Hollingsworth A. Screening for breast cancer risk in the obstetric/gynecological setting: a breast surgeon's perspective. Expert Rev Obstet Gynecol 2008;3(1):59–63.
61. Morrow M, Vogel V, Ljung BM, et al. Evaluation and management of women with an abnormal ductal lavage. J Am Coll Surg 2002;194:648–56.
62. O'Shaughnessy JA, Ljung BM, Dooley WC, et al. Ductal lavage and the clinical management of women at high risk for breast carcinoma: a commentary. Cancer 2002;94(2):292–8.
63. Hollingsworth AB, Singletary SE, Morrow M, et al. Current comprehensive assessment and management of women at increased risk for breast cancer. Am J Surg 2004;187:349–62.
64. Vogel VG. Atypia in the assessment of breast cancer risk: implications for management. Diagn Cytopathol 2004;30:151–7.
65. Kurian AW, Mills MA, Jaffee M, et al. Ductal lavage of fluid-yielding and non-fluid yielding ducts in BRCA1 and BRCA2 mutation carriers and other women at high inherited breast cancer risk. Cancer Epidemiol Biomarkers Prev 2005;14(5):1082–9.
66. Mitchell G, Antill YC, Murray W, et al. Nipple aspiration and ductal lavage in women with a germline BRCA1 or BRCA2 mutation. Breast Cancer Res 2005;7:R1122–31.
67. Carruthers CD, Chapleskie LA, Flynn MB, et al. Use of ductal lavage as a screening tool in women at high risk for developing breast carcinoma. Am J Surg 2007;194(4):463–6.
68. Loud JT, Thiebaut AC, Abati AD, et al. Ductal lavage in women from BRCA 1.2 families: is there a future for ductal lavage in women at increased genetic risk of breast cancer? Cancer Epidemiol Biomarkers Prev 2009;18(4):1243–51.
69. Higgins SA, Matloff ET, Rimm DL, et al. Patterns of reduced nipple aspirate fluid production and ductal lavage cellularity in women at high risk for breast cancer. Breast Cancer Res 2005;7:R1017–22.
70. Arun B, Valero V, Logan C, et al. Comparison of ductal lavage and random periareolar fine needle aspiration as tissue acquisition methods in early breast cancer prevention trials. Clin Cancer Res 2007;13(16):4943–8.
71. Visvanathan K, Santor D, Ali SZ, et al. The reliability of nipple aspirate and ductal lavage in women at increased risk for breast cancer—a potential tool for breast cancer risk assessment and biomarker evaluation. Cancer Epidemiol Biomarkers Prev 2007;16(5):950–5.
72. Patil DB, Lankes HA, Nayar ER, et al. Reproducibility of ductal lavage cytology and cellularity over a six month interval in high risk women. Breast Cancer Res Treat 2008;112:327–33.
73. Khan SA, Lankes HA, Patil DB, et al. Ductal lavage is an inefficient method of biomarker measurement in high-risk women. Cancer Prev Res (Phila) 2009;2(3):265–73.
74. Khan SA, Wiley EL, Rodriguez N, et al. Ductal lavage findings in women with known breast cancer undergoing mastectomy. J Natl Cancer Inst 2004;96:1510–7.
75. Fabian CJ, Kimler BF, Mayo MS, et al. Breast tissue sampling for risk assessment and prevention. Endocrine related Cancer 2005;12(2):185–213.

76. Khan SA, Baird C, Staradub VL, et al. Ductal lavage an ductoscopy: the opportunities and the limitations. Clin Breast Cancer 2002;3:185–91.
77. Ljung MB, Chew KL, Moore DH, et al. Cytology of ductal lavage fluid of the breast. Diagn Cytopathol 2004;30:143–50.
78. Fabian CJ, Kimler BF, Mayo MS. Ductal lavage for early detection—what doesn't come out in the wash? J Natl Cancer Inst 2004;96(20):1488–9.
79. Green VL, Peralta N. Use of ductal lavage among women at high risk for breast cancer followed in an indigent care resident breast clinic [abstract]. Obstet Gynecol 2004;103(Suppl 4):95S.
80. Tondre J, Nejad M, Casano A, et al. Technical enhancements to breast ductal lavage. Ann Surg Oncol 2008;15(10):2734–8.
81. Golewale NH, Bryk M, Nayar R, et al. Technical modifications of ductal lavage to improve cell yield. Breast Cancer Res Treat 2003;82(Suppl 1):S175 [abstract 1024].
82. Ghanouni P, Kurian AW, Margolia DK, et al. Ductal pattern enhancement on magnetic resonance imaging of the breast due to ductal lavage. Breast J 2007;13(3):281–6.
83. Bhathal PS, Brown RW, Lesueur GC, et al. Frequency of benign and malignant breast lesions in 207 consecutive autopsies in Australian women. Br J Cancer 1985;51:271–8.
84. Nielsen M, Thomsen JL, Primdalh S, et al. Breast cancer and atypia among young and middle-aged women: a study of 110 medicolegal autopsies. Br J Cancer 1987;56:814–9.
85. Hoogerbrugge N, Bult P, DeWidt-Levert LM, et al. High prevalence of premalignant lesions in prophylactically removed breasts from women at hereditary risk for breast cancer. J Clin Oncol 2003;21:41–5.
86. Fabian CJ, Zalles C, Kamel S, et al. Prevalence of aneuploidy, overexpressed ER, and overexpressed EGFR in random breast aspirates of women at high and low risk for breast cancer. Breast Cancer Res Treat 1994;309:263–74.
87. Ibarra-Drendall C, Wilke LG, Zalles C, et al. Reproducibility of random periareolar fine needle aspiration in a multi institutional Cancer and Leukemia Group B (CALGB) cross sectional study. Cancer Epidemiol Biomarkers Prev 2009;18(5):1379–85.
88. Fabian CJ, Kimler BF, Zalles CM, et al. Short-term breast cancer prediction by random periareolar fine-needle aspiration cytology and the Gail risk model. J Natl Cancer Inst 2000;92:1217–27.
89. Fabian CJ, Kimler BF. Breast cancer risk prediction: should nipple aspiration fluid cytology be incorporated into clinical practice? J Natl Cancer Inst 2001; 93(23):1762–3.
90. NCCN clinical practice guidelines in oncology. Breast cancer risk reduction. Available at: www.nccn.org. BRISK 3 footnote N. version1.2012. Accessed February 9, 2013.
91. Available at: www.cancer.gov/newscenter/lavage. Accessed November 4, 2009.
92. Dalessandri KM, Miike R, Wrensch MR, et al. Presented at the 31st Annual San Antonio Breast Cancer Symposium Session: Risk and Prevention: Poster Discussion 5, December 12, 2008. Available at: www.sabcs.org/ProgramSchedule/PosterSessions.asp?SessionGroupID=57. Abstract Number: 502. Title: Validation of OncoVue, a new individualized breast cancer risk estimator in the Marin County, California adolescent risk study.
93. American Cancer Society. *Cancer Facts & Figures for African Americans 2013-2014*. Atlanta (GA): American Cancer Society; 2013. Available at: http://www.cancer.org/acs/groups/content @epidemiologysurveilance/documents/document/acspc-036921.pdf. Accessed August 3, 2013.

94. Kotsopoulos J, Lubinski J, Salmena L, et al. Breastfeeding and the risk of breast cancer in the BRCA1 and BRCA2 mutation carriers. Breast Cancer Res 2012; 14(2):R42.

95. Fisher B, Dignam J, Wolmark N, et al. Tamoxifen in treatment of intraductal breast cancer: National Surgical Adjuvant Breast and Bowel Project B24 randomized controlled trial. Lancet 1999;353(9169):1993–2000.

96. Fisher B, Costantino J, Wickerham D, et al. Tamoxifen for the prevention of breast cancer: current status of the National Surgical Adjuvant Breast and Bowel Project P-1 study. J Natl Cancer Inst 2005;97:1652–62.

97. Cuzick J, Forbes J, Edwards R, et al. First results from the International Breast Cancer Intervention Study (IBIS-I): a randomized prevention trial. Lancet 2002; 360(9336):817–24.

98. Cuzick J, Forbes JF, Sestak I, et al. Long term results of tamoxifen prophylaxis for breast cancer—96 month follow up of the randomized IBIS-I trial. J Natl Cancer Inst 2007;99(4):272–82.

99. Powles J, Eeles R, Ashley S, et al. Interim analysis of the incidence of breast cancer in the royal Marsden Hospital tamoxifen randomized chemoprevention trial. Lancet 1998;352:98–101.

100. Powles TJ, Ashley S, Tidy A, et al. Twenty year follow up of the Royal Marsden randomized, double blinded tamoxifen breast cancer prevention trial. J Natl Cancer Inst 2007;99(4):283–90.

101. Veronesi U, Maisonneuve P, Sacchni V, et al. Tamoxifen for breast cancer among hysterectomized women. Lancet 2002;359:1122–4.

102. Veronesi U, Maisonneuve P, Rotmensz N, et al. Italian randomized trial among women with hysterectomy: tamoxifen and hormone dependent breast cancer in high risk women. J Natl Cancer Inst 2003;95:160–5.

103. Cuzick J, Powles T, Veronesi U, et al. Overview of the main outcomes in breast cancer prevention trials. Lancet 2003;361:296–300.

104. Cauley JA, Norton L, Lippman ET, et al. Continued breast cancer risk reduction in postmenopausal women treated with raloxifene: 43 year results from the MORE trial. Multiple outcomes of raloxifene evaluation. Breast Cancer Res Treat 2001;65:125–34.

105. Martino S, Cauley JA, Barrett-Connor E, et al. Continuing outcomes relevant to Evista: breast cancer incidence in postmenopausal osteoporotic women in a randomized trial of raloxifene. J Natl Cancer Inst 2004;96:1751–61.

106. Barrett-Connor E, Mosca L, Collins P, et al. Effect of raloxifene on cardiovascular events and breast cancer in postmenopausal women. N Engl J Med 2006;355: 125–37.

107. Vogel VG, Costantino JP, Wickerham DL, et al. Update of the national Surgical Adjuvant Breast and Bowel Project Study of Tamoxifen and Raloxifene (STAR) P2 trial: preventing breast cancer. Cancer Prev Res (Phila) 2010;3: 696–706.

108. Land SR, Wickerham DL, Costantino JR, et al. Patient-reported symptoms and quality of life during treatment of tamoxifen and raloxifene for breast cancer prevention: the NSABP Study of Tamoxifen and Raloxifene (STAR) P-2 trial. JAMA 2006;295(23):2742–51.

109. Cuzick J, DeCensi A, Banu A, et al. Preventive therapy for breast cancer: a consensus statement. Lancet 2011;12:496–503.

110. Narod SA, Brunet JS, Ghadirian P, et al. Tamoxifen and risk of contralateral breast cancer in BRCA1 and BRCA2 mutation carriers: a case control study. Hereditary Breast Cancer Clinical Study Group. Lancet 2000;356:1876–81.

111. Baum M, Budzar AU, Cuzick J, et al. Anastrozole alone or in combination with tamoxifen versus tamoxifen alone for adjuvant treatment of postmenopausal women with early breast cancer: first results of the ATAC randomized trial. Lancet 2002;359:2131–9.

112. Baum M, Budzar AU, Cuzick J, et al. Anastrozole alone or in combination with tamoxifen versus tamoxifen alone for adjuvant treatment of postmenopausal women with early breast cancer: results of the ATAC Arimidex, Tamoxifen Alone or in Combination: trial efficacy and safety update analyses. Cancer 2003;98: 1802–10.

113. Coombes RC, Hall E, Gibson LJ, et al. A randomized trial of exemestane after two to three years of tamoxifen therapy in postmenopausal women with primary breast cancer. N Engl J Med 2004;350:1081–92.

114. Goss PE, Ingle JN, Martino S, et al. A randomized trial of letrozole in postmenopausal women after five years of tamoxifen therapy for early-stage breast cancer. N Engl J Med 2003;349:1793–802.

115. Thurlimann B, Keshaviah A, Coates AS, et al. A comparison of letrozole and tamoxifen in postmenopausal women with early breast cancer. N Engl J Med 2005;353:2747–57.

116. Goss PE, Ingle JN, Ales-Martinez JE, et al. Exemestane for breast cancer prevention in postmenopausal women. N Engl J Med 2011;364:2381–91.

117. National Comprehensive Cancer Network Guidelines Version 1/2012. Breast cancer risk reduction. MS 13. Available at: http://www.nccn.org/professionals/physician_gls/f_guidelines.asp#detection. Accessed March 3, 2013.

118. Cheung AM, Tile L, Cardew S, et al. Bone density and structure in healthy postmenopausal women treated with Exemestane for the primary prevention of breast cancer: a nested substudy of the MAP 3 randomised controlled trial. Lancet Oncol 2012;13(3):275–84.

119. National Comprehensive Cancer Network Guidelines Version 1/2012. Breast cancer risk reduction. MS 15. Available at: http://www.nccn.org/professionals/physician_gls/f_guidelines.asp#detection. Accessed February 16, 2013.

120. Yang Z, Simondsen K, Kolesar J. Exemestane for primary prevention of breast cancer in postmenopausal women. Am J Health Syst Pharm 2012;69(16): 1384–8.

121. Cuzick J. Aromatase inhibitors for breast cancer prevention. J Clin Oncol 2005; 23:1636–43.

122. Singh S, Cuzick J, Mesher D, et al. Effect of baseline serum vitamin D levels on aromatase inhibitors induced musculoskeletal symptoms: results from the IBIS II chemoprevention study using anastrozole. Breast Cancer Res Treat 2012; 132(2):625–9.

123. Visvanathan K, Lippman SM, Hurley P, et al. American Society of Clinical Oncology clinical practice guideline update on the use of pharmacologic interventions including tamoxifen, raloxifene, and aromatase inhibition for breast cancer risk reduction. Gynecol Oncol 2009;115(1):132–4.

124. Zanardi S, Serrano D, Argusti A, et al. Clinical trials with retinoids for breast cancer chemoprevention. Endocr Relat Cancer 2006;13:51–68.

125. Li Y, Zhang Y, Hill J, et al. The rexinoid LG100268 prevents the development of preinvasive and invasive estrogen receptor negative tumors in MMTV erbB2 mice. Clin Cancer Res 2007;13:6224–31.

126. Khan SA, Chatterton RT, Michel N, et al. Soy isoflavone supplementation for breast cancer risk reduction: a randomized phase II trial. Cancer Prev Res (Phila) 2012;5(2):309–19.

127. Fabian CJ, Kimler BF, Zalles CM, et al. Reduction of Ki67 in benign breast tissue of high risk women with the lignin secolariciresinol diglycoside. Cancer Prev Res (Phila) 2010;3(10):1342–50.
128. Zhao YS, Zhu S, Li XW, et al. Association between NSAIDs use and breast cancer risk: a systematic review and meta-analysis. Breast Cancer Res Treat 2009; 117:141–50.
129. Mukherjee D, Missen SE, Topol EJ. Risk of cardiovascular events associated with selective COX 2 inhibitors. JAMA 2001;286(8):954–9.
130. Dalessandri KM, Miike R, Wiencke JK, et al. Vitamin D receptor polymorphisms and breast cancer risk in a high incidence population: a pilot study. J Am Coll Surg 2011;215(5):652–7.
131. Vogel VG. Can statin therapy reduce the risk of breast cancer? J Clin Oncol 2005;23:8553–5.
132. Browning DR, Martin RM. Statins and risk of cancer: a systematic review and metaanalysis. Int J Cancer 2007;120:833–43.
133. Bopnovas S, Filioussi K, Tsavaris N, et al. Use of statins and breast cancer: a meta-analysis of seven randomized clinical trials and nine observational studies. J Clin Oncol 2005;23:8606–12.
134. Baigent C, Keech A, Kearney PM, et al. Efficacy and safety of cholesterol lowering treatment: prospective meta analysis of data from 90,056 participants in 14 randomised trials of statins. Lancet 2005;366:1267–78.
135. Dale KM, Coleman CI, Henyan NN, et al. Statins and cancer risk: a metaanalysis. JAMA 2006;295:74–80.
136. Kumar AS, Benz CC, Shim V, et al. Estrogen receptor negative breast cancer is less likely to arise among lipophilic statin users. Cancer Epidemiol Biomarkers Prev 2008;17(5):1028–33.
137. Garwood ER, Kumar AS, Baehner FL, et al. Fluvastatin reduces proliferation and increases apoptosis in women with high grade breast cancer. Breast Cancer Res Treat 2010;119(1):137–44.
138. Cummings SR, Ettinger B, Delmas PD, et al. The effects of tibolone in older postmenopausal women. N Engl J Med 2008;359:697–708.
139. Cummings SR, McClung M, Reginster J, et al. Arzoxifene for prevention of fractures and invasive breast cancer in postmenopausal women. J Bone Miner Res 2011;26(2):397–404.
140. Cummings SR, Ensrud K, Delmas PE, et al. Lasofoxifene in postmenopausal women with osteoporosis. N Engl J Med 2010;362:686–96.
141. Bodmer M, Meier C, Krahenbuhl S, et al. Long term metformin use is associated with decreased risk of breast cancer. Diabetes Care 2010;33:1304–8.
142. Bosco JL, Antosen S, Sorensen HT, et al. Metformin and incident breast cancer among diabetic women: a population based case control study in Denmark. Cancer Epidemiol Biomarkers Prev 2011;20:101–11.
143. Rennert G, Pinchev M, Rennert HS. Use of bisphosphonates and risk of postmenopausal breast cancer. J Clin Oncol 2010;28:3577–81.
144. Chlebowski RT, Chen Z, Cauley JA, et al. Oral bisphosphonate use and breast cancer incidence in postmenopausal women. J Clin Oncol 2010;28: 3582–90.
145. Ibarra-Drendall C, Troch MM, Barry WT, et al. Pilot and feasibility study: prospective proteomic profiling of mammary epithelial cells from high risk women provides evidence of activation of pro survival pathways. Breast Cancer Res Treat 2012;132(2):487–98.

146. Burch PA, Breen JK, Budkner JC, et al. Priming tissue specific cellular immunity in a Phase I trial of autologous dendritic cells for prostate cancer. Clin Cancer Res 2000;6(6):2175–82.

147. Rosenberg SA, Yang JC, Restifo NP. Cancer immunotherapy: moving beyond current vaccines. Nat Med 2004;10(9):909–15.

148. Mittendorf EA, Altrash G, Xiao H, et al. Breast cancer vaccines: ongoing National Cancer Institute-registered clinical trials. Expert Rev Vaccines 2011; 10(6):755–74.

Obstetrics and Gynecology Physicians

A Critical Part of the Health Care Team for Women with Newly Diagnosed Breast Cancer

James Mullet, MD*, Catherine Hagan-Aylor, BA, BSN, MSN, CBCN

KEYWORDS

- Diagnosis • Map features • Chronology • Interdisciplinary conference
- OB/GYN physician

KEY POINTS

- This article will help obstetrics and gynecology (OB/GYN) physicians assure women that the tests being performed to map the individual features of newly diagnosed breast cancer follow a predictable and organized process.
- This article reviews general concepts about breast cancer. Regular attendance at interdisciplinary breast cancer conferences will help OB/GYN physicians develop the required knowledge to counsel women with new breast cancer.
- This article explains that, in many cases, the OB/GYN physician can work with the breast imager to reassure the patient of a good outcome based on the diagnostic mammography features.

INTRODUCTION

A woman with newly diagnosed breast cancer will benefit from reassurance from her obstetrics and gynecology (OB/GYN) physician. This is particularly true if the OB/GYN physician understands and communicates the chronology and meaning of the multiple tests being performed to map the individual features of a woman's breast cancer before she meets with the breast cancer specialists who will treat her.

THE OB/GYN PHYSICIAN ROLE

As treatment of breast cancer becomes more individualized, depending on both the extent of disease and individual tumor features, the American College of Obstetricians

Disclosures: The authors have nothing to disclose.
Department of Radiology, Carilion Clinic Breast Care Center, 102 Highland Avenue, Suite 202, Roanoke, VA 24013, USA
* Corresponding author.
E-mail address: jgmullet@carilionclinic.org

Obstet Gynecol Clin N Am 40 (2013) 551–558
http://dx.doi.org/10.1016/j.ogc.2013.05.008   obgyn.theclinics.com
0889-8545/13/$ – see front matter © 2013 Elsevier Inc. All rights reserved.

and Gynecologists reports that it is increasingly important for women's health care providers to have an understanding of breast cancer.[1] This article focuses on the initial period after the detection and diagnosis of a woman's breast cancer, before her visit to the breast cancer specialists who will treat her. Coordinated and consistent communication to the patient requires that the OB/GYN physician and other members of the health care team understand their roles and are knowledgeable about breast cancer diagnosis and therapy, and this article suggests methods for OB/GYN physicians to improve these skills.

Most OB/GYN physicians assist their patients at the time of diagnosis of breast cancer, but few take part in therapy planning.[2] Although a woman often understands the need to wait a few days to have a comprehensive discussion with the breast cancer specialists who will treat her, those days of waiting can be very difficult. During this time, the patient's OB/GYN physician can assure her that the tests being performed to map the individual features of her breast cancer follow a predictable and organized process. The OB/GYN physician can provide the contact information for specific breast care team members for guidance and support. Each breast care program may evolve slightly differently, but the role of the breast imager, nurse navigator, and OB/GYN physician should be clarified for that program.

At the time of diagnosis, the patient's interest in learning specific information about her cancer must be assessed. The provision of information should match the wishes of the individual patient. Most patients who want information want as much as possible (both good and bad) as it becomes available.[3] The OB/GYN physician can provide the patient with the chronologic sequence of the ongoing tests and explain what they mean (**Fig. 1**). The summary shown in **Fig. 1** is intended to be a guide for the OB/GYN physician and a communication tool for patient discussion. For example, based on this guide, the patient would know that the clinical staging would not be available until the previous steps were complete.

This period can be a fruitful time of information gathering and preparation for the patient. The information she is given can guide her Internet queries. Because most breast cancers have a good prognosis, her search may generally be reassuring. The OB/GYN can caution her, however, that information on the Internet or through social media can be inaccurate or misleading. Peer reviewed and nationally recognized Web sites can be suggested, as noted in the article by Mitchell and colleagues elsewhere in this issue.

GENERAL CONCEPTS ABOUT BREAST CANCER

Breast cancer arises from the normal epithelial cells that line the inner surface of the milk-producing and milk-transporting structures of the breast. Most breast cancer arises in the tiny tubules (acini) of the milk-producing structures (lobules). Less commonly, breast cancer arises in the larger milk-transporting ducts. Breast cancer cells differ from normal cells because they have some critical genetic errors that signal them to lose normal control of division and function.

The possible combinations of important features of each individual breast cancer are virtually limitless. Each individual diagnostic test "sees" some specific features of the individual patient's cancer through its lens. Each diagnostic test can clarify only to some degree the nature of part of the cancer.

CARCINOMA IN SITU OF THE BREAST

In the era of mammography screening, approximately 25% of breast cancers are confined to within acini of the milk-producing lobules or within the larger ducts,

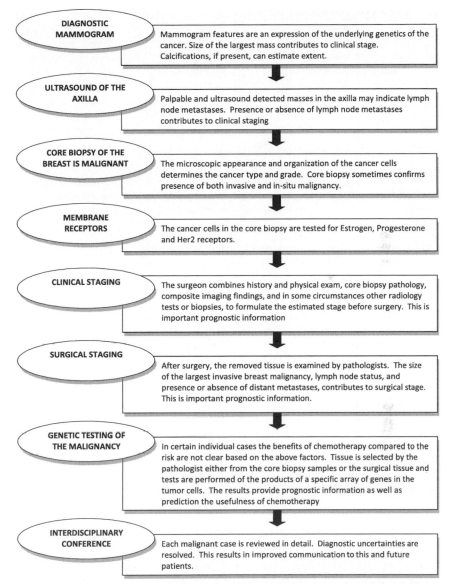

Fig. 1. Important features of a woman's individual breast cancer are discovered in this chronologic order.

and no invasive lump of cancer cells is present; these are carcinoma in situ (**Fig. 2**). These cases are usually discovered through calcifications detected on the mammogram.

INVASIVE BREAST CANCER

In the remainder of cases, an invasive component of cancer is present, either with or without carcinoma in situ. Most breast cancers (76%) are a combination of invasive

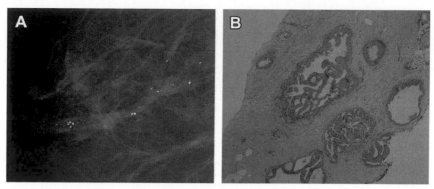

Fig. 2. Carcinoma in situ in large a duct detected by mammogram calcifications (A) with corresponding cribriform intermediate nuclear grade carcinoma in situ (B) at histology (hematoxylin-eosin).

and in situ cancer.[4] The invasive cancer can be one mass (58%), multiple masses (38%), or, less commonly, a sheet-like or spider's web–like mass (**Fig. 3**).[5]

EXTENT OF BREAST CANCER

The extent of breast cancer is defined as the measured pathology (including both invasive and in situ) from one end to the other of the malignant structures. Estimation of extent through imaging and the location of cancer are very important in surgical planning (**Fig. 4**). If the extent of breast cancer is too great, breast conservation surgery will not be possible.

Early breast cancers are often just as extensive as advanced cancers.[6] Although some breast cancers arise in a "ball" of cancer cells, most arise from a field of tissue. The exact mechanism remains largely unclear.[7] Extensive breast cancers may arise from a cancer progenitor cell. Its progeny populate a field of the breast.[8] A central component of the treatment planning for breast cancer is full knowledge of the extent of disease and its biologic features.[9]

PATHOLOGY GRADE OF BREAST CANCER

The pathologist assesses the microscopic appearance and organization of the cancer cells to determine the type and grade of the breast cancer (**Fig. 5**).

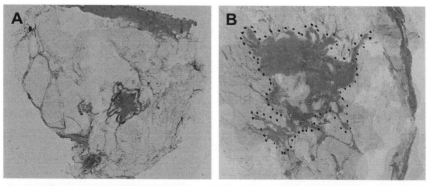

Fig. 3. Multifocal (A) and diffuse (spider's web–like or sheet-like) pattern of malignancy (B). (hematoxylin-eosin).

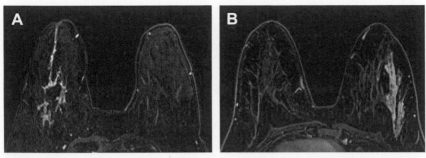

Fig. 4. Extent is the measure of both in situ and invasive malignancy. Extensive mostly in situ malignancy shown on magnetic resonance imaging (MRI) (*B*). Extensive diffuse invasive malignancy shown on MRI (*A*). (Gadolinium enhancement).

MEMBRANE RECEPTORS

Most breast cancers retain receptors on their membranes for estrogen and progesterone (**Fig. 6**). In some cancers these receptors are lost. In some cases growth receptors (such as HER2) may be amplified. The receptor information is important when planning patient-specific chemotherapy or hormonal therapy.

GENETIC TESTING OF BREAST CANCER

The information coded by some of the genes in breast cancer cells can be studied by special tests.[10] An array of genes can be tested to predict prognosis and whether chemotherapy would help reduce the chances of fatality from that cancer.[11]

STAGING OF BREAST CANCER

Sometimes cancer cells have spread to other sites at the time of diagnosis. Sometimes the cancer cells spread through the lymphatic system and deposit in the axillary lymph nodes. Sometimes the cancer cells spread through the bloodstream to distant locations (**Fig. 7**). Lymphatic or distant metastases are a component of staging. Staging is a summary of tumor size and lymph node or distant disease status,[12] and is a very important prognostic and therapy planning tool.

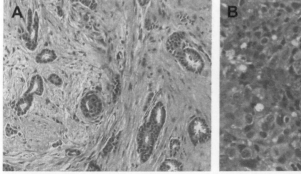
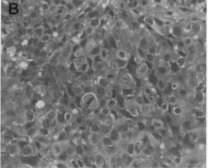

Fig. 5. Low-grade invasive breast cancer (*A*). High-grade invasive breast cancer (*B*). (hematoxylin-eosin).

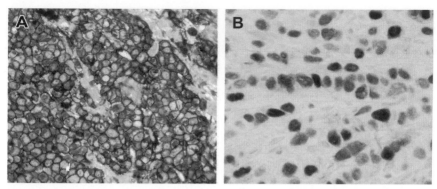

Fig. 6. Cancer cell membranes stain positive for HER2 receptors (Immunohistochemical stain for HER2 receptors) (*A*) and nuclear stain is positive for estrogen receptors (Immunohistochemical stain for estrogen receptors) (*B*).

USING THE PROGNOSTIC VALUE OF THE MAMMOGRAM

The mammogram can provide an excellent prognostic value for many patients. Mammography screening detects a large number of in situ and small invasive cancers measuring less than 15 mm. This group can represent more than 50% of all cancer in practices with active screening programs. Of this group, the stellate/spiculated masses without calcifications constitute the largest category and have an excellent long term outcome (**Fig. 8**).[13]

THE INTERDISCIPLINARY BREAST CANCER CONFERENCE

Comprehensive breast cancer programs have regular interdisciplinary conferences in which the results of the diagnostic tests of each patient with newly diagnosed breast cancer are reviewed. Diagnostic uncertainties are resolved through correlation of imaging and pathology studies, and staging is established. The therapeutic plan for each patient is outlined and discussed. OB/GYN physicians have the opportunity to participate in this discussion and understand the care plan for their patients. Regular attendance at this conference will help OB/GYN physicians increase the knowledge required to counsel current and future patients.

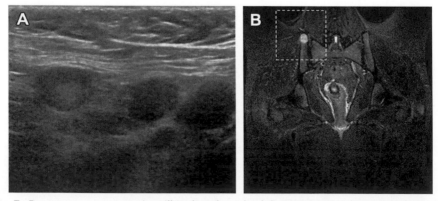

Fig. 7. Breast cancer metastatic axillary lymph nodes (*A*). Breast cancer bone metastasis (*B*).

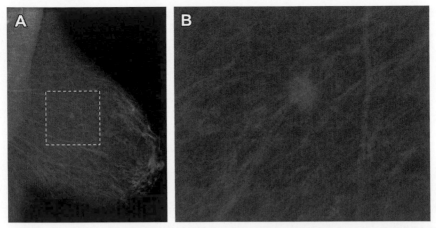

Fig. 8. Small stellate/spiculated masses without calcifications are often detected by screening mammography (*A*). A magnification view confirms the stellate/spiculated pattern (*B*).

SUMMARY

Most OB/GYN physicians assist their patients at the time of a new breast cancer diagnosis. Although the diagnosis and therapy planning is an ongoing process, the OB/GYN physician can assure a woman that the tests being performed to map the individual features of her breast cancer follow a predictable and organized process. OB/GYN physicians can provide patients with information about the chronology of the diagnostic process. In many cases, it is appropriate to confidently reassure the patient of a good outcome based on the diagnostic mammography features. Regular attendance at interdisciplinary breast cancer conferences will help OB/GYN physicians develop the required knowledge to counsel women with newly diagnosed breast cancer.

REFERENCES

1. Committee on Practice Bulletins-Gynecology. Management of gynecologic issues in women with breast cancer. Obstet Gynecol 2012;119(3):666–82.
2. Galand-Desme S, Milliat-Guittard L, Letrilliart L, et al. Role of gynecologists in the care of women with breast cancer. J Gynecol Obstet Biol Reprod (Paris) 2005; 34(8):775–80 [in French].
3. Sowden AJ, Forbes C, Entwistle V, et al. Informing, communicating and sharing decisions with people who have cancer. Qual Health Care 2001;10:193–6.
4. Tot T. Clinical relevance of the distribution of the lesions in 500 consecutive breast cancer cases documented in large-format histologic sections. Cancer 2007; 110(11):2551–60.
5. Tot T. Axillary lymph node status in unifocal, multifocal, and diffuse breast carcinomas: differences are related to macrometastatic disease. Ann Surg Oncol 2012;19(11):3395–401.
6. Holland R, Veling SH, Mravunac M, et al. Histologic multifocality of Tis, T1-2 breast carcinomas: implications for clinical trials of breast-conserving surgery. Cancer 1985;56(5):979–90.
7. Heaphy CM, Griffith JK, Bisoffi M. Mammary field cancerization: molecular evidence and clinical importance. Breast Cancer Res Treat 2009;118(2): 229–39.

8. Agelopoulos K, Buerger H, Brandt B. Allelic imbalances of the egfr gene as key events in breast cancer progression – the concept of committed progenitor cells. Curr Cancer Drug Targets 2008;8(5):431–45.

9. Theriault RL, Carlson RW, Allred C, et al. NCCN Clinical Practice Guidelines: Breast Cancer. Version 3. February 17, 2013. Available at: www.nccn.org.

10. Paik S, Shak S, Tang G, et al. A multigene assay to predict recurrence of tamoxifen-treated, node-negative breast cancer. N Engl J Med 2004;351: 2817–26.

11. Paik S, Tang G, Shak S, et al. Gene expression and benefit of chemotherapy in women with node-negative, estrogen receptor-positive breast cancer. J Clin Oncol 2006;24(23):3726–34.

12. Edge SB, Byrd DR, Compton CC, et al. AJCC cancer staging manual. 7th edition. New York: Springer; 2010.

13. Tabar L, Tucker L, Davenport RR, et al. The use of mammographic tumour feature significantly improves prediction of breast cancers smaller than 15 mm: a reproducibility study from two comprehensive breast centres. Memo 2011;4(3): 149–57.

Breast Cancer in Pregnancy

Iris Krishna, MD, MPH*, Michael Lindsay, MD, MPH

KEYWORDS

- Breast cancer • Pregnancy • Diagnosis • Chemotherapy • Prenatal care

KEY POINTS

- Breast cancer is one of the most common cancers to occur during pregnancy and, as more women delay childbearing, the incidence of breast cancer in pregnancy is expected to increase.
- Pregnancy-associated breast cancer is defined as breast cancer diagnosed during pregnancy or in the first postpartum year.
- Diagnosis of breast cancer in pregnant women is difficult due to physiologic changes that occur during pregnancy. It usually presents as a palpable mass, and any mass present for more than 2 weeks should be evaluated further via imaging and biopsy.
- The treatment of breast cancer during pregnancy should follow the guidelines recommended for nonpregnant women. Surgery can be performed safely in any stage of pregnancy with minimal complications. Anthracycline-based chemotherapy administered during the second and third trimesters is the regimen of choice. Radiation therapy is delayed until the postpartum period.
- Timing of delivery should take into account maternal status, need for further therapy, and expected fetal outcome. Iatrogenic preterm delivery should be avoided.

INTRODUCTION

Breast cancer is one of the most common malignancies occurring in women. The Centers for Disease Control and Prevention estimates that the rate of breast cancer is approximately 123 per 100,000 women.[1] Pregnancy-associated breast cancer is defined as breast cancer diagnosed during pregnancy or in the first postpartum year. It is the most common cause of invasive cancer in pregnant women and it is estimated that the rate of breast cancer in pregnancy is 6.5 per 100,000 live births.[2,3] Women over the age of 35 are at greatest risk of breast cancer in pregnancy and, as more women delay childbearing, the incidence of breast cancer in pregnancy is

Disclosures: The authors declare no financial relationships or conflicts of interest.
Department of Gynecology and Obstetrics, Division of Maternal-Fetal Medicine, Emory University School of Medicine, 69 Jesse Hill Jr Drive, Southeast, Atlanta, GA 30303, USA
* Corresponding author.
E-mail address: iris.krishna@emory.edu

Obstet Gynecol Clin N Am 40 (2013) 559–571
http://dx.doi.org/10.1016/j.ogc.2013.05.006
0889-8545/13/$ – see front matter © 2013 Elsevier Inc. All rights reserved.

obgyn.theclinics.com

expected to increase.[3] Pregnant women with breast cancer present a unique challenge to clinicians and care should involve a multidisciplinary team approach, including an obstetrician, maternal-fetal medicine specialist, medical oncologist, surgical oncologist, geneticist, and neonatologist.

CLINICAL PRESENTATION

Diagnosis of breast cancer in pregnant women is difficult owing to the physiologic changes of the breast that occur during pregnancy, which include hypertrophy, engorgement, nodularity, and discharge.[4] As a result of these physiologic changes, there is often a delay in diagnosis of breast cancer, with pregnant women often diagnosed in advanced stages and having poorer prognosis on presentation than nonpregnant women.[5–9]

The typical presentation of breast cancer in both pregnant and nonpregnant women is a painless, palpable mass.[4] It is recommended that a thorough breast examination be performed at the first prenatal visit. Women should be counseled on breast self-awareness and encouraged to notify their providers of any breast changes. Most breast masses in pregnancy are benign. The differential diagnosis of breast masses in pregnancy includes lactating adenoma, fibrocystic disease, milk retention cyst, abscess, lipoma, and hamartoma.[4,10–12] It is important for clinicians to have a high index of suspicion for malignancy, and a mass present for more than 2 weeks should be evaluated further via imaging and biopsy. The evaluation of a breast mass via imaging or biopsy should not be delayed due to pregnancy.

DIAGNOSIS
Imaging

Mammography and breast ultrasonography are the most common imaging modalities used in evaluating a suspicious breast and/or axillary mass in pregnancy, with breast ultrasonography the preferred modality. Radiologic detection and evaluation of breast masses in pregnancy can be difficult because pregnancy breast changes may increase breast density compromising the sensitivity of breast imaging with mammography and ultrasound. Studies suggest that the sensitivity of breast imaging in pregnancy seems similar to that in nonpregnant women.[13,14] Yang and colleagues[13] retrospectively reviewed mammogram and ultrasound images among women with breast cancer and found that breast cancer was visible mammographically in 90% of cases and via ultrasonography in 100% of cases. The authors noted that their findings may have been influenced by the fact that the majority of patients had more advanced stage breast cancer.

Mammography performed during pregnancy with adequate abdominal shielding poses minimal risk to the fetus.[10–12] Average fetal radiation exposure due to a mammogram is estimated at 0.4 mrad (4 μGy), which is less than the 5 rad (50 mGy) level known to be associated with fetal malformations.[10–12] Mammography is capable of characterizing a breast mass, breast density, and malignant calcifications and should be used when breast cancer is suspected.[10,13]

Ultrasonography is useful in determining if a breast mass is cystic or solid and can characterize the mass margins, echo pattern, shape, vascularity, presence of calcifications, and acoustic features.[13] Ultrasonography can also be used for assessment of the regional lymph node basins: axillary, infraclavicular, internal mammary, and supraclavicular regions. Yang and colleagues[13] demonstrated that ultrasonography could identify additional breast tumors not identified with mammography. In their series, ultrasonography led to a diagnosis of multicentric breast cancers, enabled accurate regional staging of the cancers that facilitated the appropriate treatment plan, and was a useful modality in the assessment of response of pregnant women to neoadjuvant chemotherapy by measurements of tumor shrinkage.

Mammography and ultrasound have demonstrated a complementary role in the diagnosis of breast cancer; therefore, it is reasonable to initiate evaluation of a breast mass during pregnancy with ultrasonography, if breast cancer is suspected, further evaluation for bilateral and multicentric disease via mammography should be initiated (**Fig. 1**).[13,15]

MRI requires the use of gadolinium for best imaging of the breast. Currently, there are insufficient data regarding the safety of gadolinium in pregnancy; therefore, use of gadolinium-enhanced MRI should be reserved until the postpartum period.[11]

Biopsy

According to the National Comprehensive Cancer Network (NCCN), fine-needle aspiration can be used to evaluate a suspicious breast mass and lymph nodes.[15] Core needle biopsy, however, is the preferred technique for diagnosis of breast cancer (see **Fig. 1**). A core biopsy provides sufficient tissue for histologic confirmation of breast cancer, determination of hormone receptor status, and HER2 analyses. A pathologist should be notified that the biopsy is from a pregnant patient because false-positive cytologic findings can occur due to the highly proliferative state of the breast in pregnancy.[11,15]

Staging

Once breast cancer is diagnosed, a complete staging evaluation should be performed. Staging for breast cancer in pregnancy follows the TNM staging system of the American Joint Committee on Cancer.[15] Staging studies should be tailored to minimize radiation exposure to the fetus.[15]

Breast cancer most commonly metastasizes to the lungs, liver, and bone. Chest radiograph with abdominal shielding, liver ultrasonography, and noncontrast skeletal MRI should be performed to investigate for metastatic disease.[12] CT and bone scans are not recommended for staging because of concerns for radiation exposure to the developing fetus.[10,11] Consideration should also be given to performance of baseline laboratory studies (liver and renal function and complete blood count with differential) and echocardiogram before initiation of systemic treatment, especially if anthracycline-based chemotherapy is planned.[11]

A baseline obstetric evaluation should also be performed with an assessment of baseline comorbidities that may additionally complicate pregnancy, such as hypertension and diabetes, as well as prior pregnancy complications, such as preterm labor. An ultrasound confirming dates and fetal development should be obtained to provide adequate counseling regarding pregnancy management.

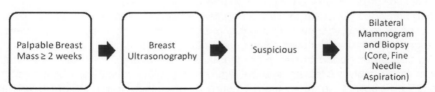

Fig. 1. Evaluation of a breast mass in pregnancy.

Pathology

The predominant histology of pregnancy-associated breast cancer is invasive ductal carcinoma.[6,10] Most of these breast cancers, compared with nonpregnant women, are diagnosed in advanced stages with large, high-grade tumors with nodal involvement, lymphovascular invasion, and hormone receptor–negative status.[6,7,10] Middleton and colleagues[6] reviewed immunohistochemical evaluation of women with pregnancy-associated breast cancer (n = 38). They found that of the 25 women tested for hormone receptor status, 7 (28%) of the tumors were estrogen receptor (ER) positive, 6 (24%) were progesterone receptor (PR) positive, and 4 (16%) were both ER/PR positive. These percentages are slightly lower than those found in age-matched nonpregnant women. These findings must be interpreted with caution because hormone-positive disease is age related and seen more often in postmenopausal women. Additionally, high levels of circulating estrogen and progesterone in pregnancy may bind all the hormone receptor sites, resulting in artificial negative receptor status in hormone binding assays; therefore, immunohistochemical evaluation should be performed to assess hormone receptor status.[4,6] These investigators found that percentage of HER2-positive tumors (n = 7, 28%) was similar to that for nonpregnant breast cancer patients.[6] Overall, it seems that the histopathologic and immunohistochemical findings among pregnant women with breast cancer are similar to those of nonpregnant women with breast cancer in the same age group. It is more likely that age at diagnosis rather than pregnancy determines the biologic features of breast cancer.[10] Given young age at diagnosis of pregnant women with breast cancer, BRCA testing should be considered.

TREATMENT

The treatment of breast cancer during pregnancy should closely follow the guidelines recommended for nonpregnant women. Therapeutic decisions should be individualized, taking into consideration the gestational age at diagnosis, stage of the disease, and preferences of patient and family (**Figs. 2–4**).

Surgery

Surgery is the first-line treatment of pregnancy-associated breast cancer. Surgery can be performed safely in any stage of pregnancy with minimal complications, such as infection and breast hematomas.[16,17] Surgeons may prefer to wait until after the first trimester because the risk of a spontaneous abortion is highest in the first trimester. It has been reported, however, that women who undergo surgery for breast cancer in the first trimester do not seem to have a higher rate of spontaneous loss compared with the general population.[16] Both mastectomy and breast-conserving surgery with axillary lymph node dissection are options.[15] Mastectomy may be preferred because follow-up breast radiation therapy is typically not warranted. After breast-conserving surgery, radiation therapy is standard. In pregnant women, radiation therapy is preferably delayed until the postpartum period. According to the NCCN guidelines, breast-conserving surgery is possible if radiation therapy can be delayed until the postpartum period and does not seem to have a negative impact on survival.[15] If breast reconstruction is desired, it should be delayed until after delivery because of the inherent changes that occur in the unaffected breast after pregnancy.[12]

Sentinel lymph node biopsies in pregnancy are controversial.[18,19] A sentinel lymph node biopsy involves injecting blue dye (eg, isosulfan blue or methylene blue) and/or a radiolabeled colloid (eg, technetium Tc 99m sulfur colloid) at the site of the primary tumor, with subsequent identification of the first draining node.[19] The aim of this

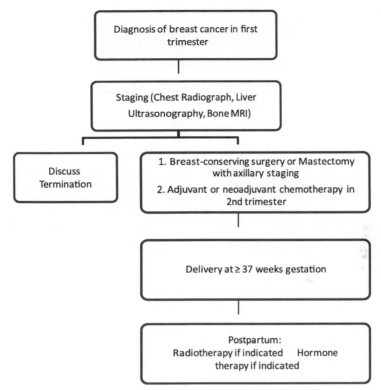

Fig. 2. Management of breast cancer diagnosed in the first trimester.

procedure is to provide staging information and to determine the need for axillary lymph node dissection. There are few data on its safety and efficacy in pregnant women.[16,18,19] Keleher and colleagues[19] estimated that the maximum absorbed dose of radiation to a fetus from a sentinel node biopsy using technetium Tc 99m sulfur colloid is approximately 0.43 rad (4.3 mGy), which is well below the radiation exposure from other nuclear medicine procedures cautiously used in pregnant women (eg, ventilation-perfusion lung scanning and venography). In a study of maternal and fetal outcomes from breast cancer by Cardonick and colleagues,[16] sentinel lymph node biopsy was performed in 30 patients, with the majority performed in the first trimester (n = 17); 9 (30%) had adverse pregnancy outcomes, 2 miscarriages occurred in the first trimester, 3 children had a birthweight less than 10% for gestational age at delivery, 2 children had complications related to prematurity, and 2 children were born with malformations.[16] Isosulfan blue or methylene blue dye mapping is not recommended in pregnant women because anaphylaxis has been observed with its use.[10] At this time, there is limited information regarding sentinel lymph node biopsies among pregnant women, but technetium-based identification has been performed successfully. Decisions related to its use should be individualized.[15]

Chemotherapy

Chemotherapy should be administered after the first trimester and can be adjuvant or neoadjuvant. Most chemotherapy agents have been categorized by the US Food and

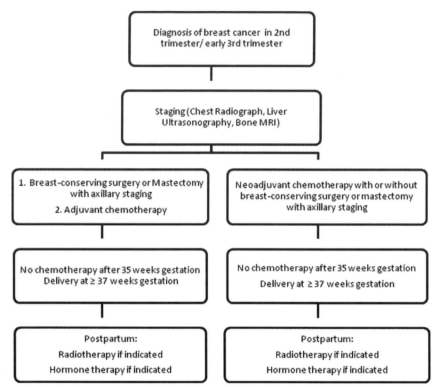

Fig. 3. Management of breast cancer diagnosed in the second trimester/early third trimester.

Drug administration as category D or X, indicating that teratogenic effects have occurred in humans but benefits in certain situations may make the use of the drug acceptable despite its risks.[4] The reported fetal malformation rate among those exposed to chemotherapy in second and third trimester is approximately 3.8%, which is not higher than that reported in the general population.[16] The available data on chemotherapy in pregnancy are limited and based on case reports, case series, and retrospective registries.

Anthracyclines

Anthracycline-based chemotherapy, doxorubicin and cyclophosphamide (AC regimen) or 5-fluorouracil, doxorubicin, and cyclophosphamide (FAC regimen), administered during the second and third trimesters is the most common regimen reported for treatment of pregnancy-associated breast cancer. Hahn and colleagues[20] have reported the largest prospective series of breast cancer patients treated with systemic chemotherapy (FAC) in pregnancy in the adjuvant or neoadjuvant setting (n = 57). At median follow-up duration of 38.5 months (range 1.0–189.0 months), 40 (70%) are alive and disease-free, 3 (5%) had a recurrent breast cancer, 12 (21%) died from breast cancer, 1 (1.7%) died from other causes, and 1 (1.7%) was lost to follow-up. All women delivered live births, with a mean gestational age of 37 weeks and average birthweight of 2890 g. Among the children exposed to chemotherapy in utero (n = 40), 3 had congenital malformations (7.5%). On short-term follow-up, the children are

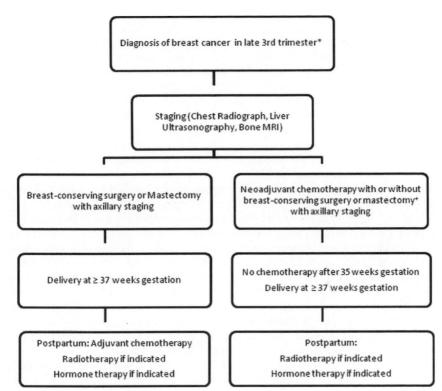

Fig. 4. Management of breast cancer diagnosed in the late third trimester. * If diagnosed ≥35 weeks, consider delivery and postpartum staging and treatment. + Surgery may be delayed until after delivery.

healthy and those in school are doing well with the exception of 2, who have special educational needs. The investigators note that one limitation of their study is that they did not have complete data on children exposed to chemotherapy due to loss to follow-up.[20]

Cardonick and colleagues[16] reported maternal and fetal outcomes among a voluntary registry of 130 women diagnosed with breast cancer in pregnancy, with the majority of patients followed prospectively. Chemotherapy was given to 104 (80%) cases and the majority of patients (69%) received doxorubicin and cyclophosphamide. Other regimens included 5-fluorouracil, doxorubicin, and cyclophosphamide; 5-fluorouracil, epirubicin, and cyclophosphamide; and doxorubicin or vinorelbine alone; several included taxanes. The most common maternal side effects included neutropenia, mouth ulcers, anaphylaxis, constipation, tachycardia, and arm cellulitis. Birthweight less than the 10% for gestational age was reported among 8 women (7.6%) who received chemotherapy. Birth defects were reported in 4 cases (3.8%) and other fetal complications were documented in 19 cases (18.2%). One neonate was diagnosed with a systematic autoimmune disorder, resulting in demise at 13 months of age. Limitations of this study include the inherent risks in collecting information through a voluntary registry, such as selection bias.[16]

Overall, based on these data, it seems that anthracycline-based chemotherapy in the second and third trimesters can be given with acceptable risk to the developing fetus.

Taxanes

There are few data on the use of taxanes during pregnancy.[21,22] Most of the data are derived from case series that include both breast and gynecologic cancers. A retrospective cohort study by Cardonick and colleagues[21] compared maternal and neonatal outcomes among women with breast or ovarian cancer who received taxanes and those who did not receive taxanes during pregnancy as identified from a voluntary registry. In this small cohort, birthweight, gestational age at delivery, growth restriction, congenital anomalies, and incidence of maternal and neonatal neutropenia were not statistically significant between women who did (n = 15) and did not (n = 114) receive taxane therapy. The investigators concluded that taxane-based chemotherapy does not seem to increase the risk of fetal or maternal complications compared with conventional therapy.[21] Study findings should be interpreted with caution, however, due to the small study size.

Mir and colleagues[22] published a systematic review of taxane use in pregnancy; 23 publications were identified describing 40 women and 42 neonates. Paclitaxel was administered in 21 cases, docetaxel in 16, and both drugs in 3 cases. The only malformation reported was pyloric stenosis in a neonate whose mother received multiagent chemotherapy along with taxanes. In 2 cases, patients exposed to paclitaxel delivered neonates at 30 and 32 weeks who subsequently developed acute respiratory distress, possibly related to prematurity, and required neonatal intensive care.[22] The investigators thought that although taxanes seem feasible in the second and third trimesters with a favorable toxicity profile, their results should be interpreted with caution based on the methodological bias associated with the data collection.[22]

Currently, the data on taxane use do not demonstrate any significant neonatal or maternal effect and may be considered an option for pregnant patients. Given the limited data, however, use should be individualized in appropriately counseled women.

Dose-Dense Chemotherapy

Among women with hormone receptor–negative breast cancer, dose-dense chemotherapy regimens have demonstrated improved disease-free survival.[23] Cardonick and colleagues[24] recently published a retrospective cohort from a voluntary registry where 10 pregnant women who received chemotherapy every 2 weeks (dose dense) were compared with 99 pregnant women who received chemotherapy with at least 3-week intervals (conventional chemotherapy). All chemotherapy was initiated after the first trimester. Birthweight, gestational age at delivery, rate of growth restriction, congenital anomalies, and incidence of maternal and neonatal neutropenia were not statistically different between the 2 groups. The incidence of birth defects in both groups (3.6%) was not higher than the baseline 3% prevalence in the general population. The overall 3.5-year survival was similar in both groups (90% vs 86%, $P>.99$, for dose-dense and conventional chemotherapy groups, respectively). The rate of spontaneous preterm birth or preterm premature rupture of membranes was 30% for the dose-dense and 17% for the conventional chemotherapy groups ($P = .188$). One neonate in the dose-dense group experienced transient neutropenia without long-term sequelae. In this small cohort, dose-dense chemotherapy did not seem to increase the risk of fetal or maternal complications. The small number of patients, lack of randomization, and lack of power, however, limit this study.[24]

Currently the data on dose-dense chemotherapeutic agents in pregnancy are limited and need additional investigation.

Trastuzumab

Trastuzumab has been established as the treatment of choice for HER2- positive breast cancer. Its use in pregnancy is associated with a high incidence of oligohydramnios when it is used beyond the first trimester. According to NCCN guidelines, its use is contraindicated in pregnancy.[15] Zagouri and colleagues[25] recently performed a systematic review and meta-analysis of trastuzumab administration in pregnancy; 17 studies were included in the meta-analysis and the main adverse event was oligohydramnios (61.1%). All children exposed to trastuzumab exclusively in the first trimester were completely healthy at birth. There was a trend of increased incidence of oligohydramnios with duration of treatment, and oligohydramnios was reversible when the agent was stopped, with good outcomes observed in the majority of patients. In general, trastuzumab should not be administered during pregnancy. In selected cases, however, where the agent may be urgently needed, it is best administered for short duration, with careful observation of amniotic fluid, fetal growth, and kidney function; in cases of oligohydramnios, the agent should be immediately discontinued.[25]

Hormone Therapy

Therapy with tamoxifen or other selective ER modulators in women with hormone receptor–positive breast cancer is deferred until after delivery.[15] Tamoxifen has the potential to disturb the hormonal environment and has been associated with birth defects, such as craniofacial malformations and ambiguous genitalia.[4,12,26]

Supportive Care

Supportive treatment of chemotherapy can be given according to general recommendations. Antiemetic agents, such as ondansetron (category B) or promethazine (category C), are routinely given in the treatment of hyperemesis gravidarum and considered safe in pregnancy. Corticosteroids can also be used for the treatment of nausea and vomiting; however, there is an association between first-trimester exposure to corticosteroids and cleft palate; therefore, its use should be restricted to after the first trimester.[27] Methylprednisolone (category C) and hydrocortisone (category C) are the preferred corticosteroids because they do not cross the placenta. Granulocyte colony-stimulating growth factor (category C) and erythropoietin (category C) have been safely administered in pregnant patients.[4]

Radiation Therapy

Radiation therapy is generally avoided during pregnancy because of the risks associated with fetal exposure to radiation.[10–12,15] It should be delayed whenever possible until the postpartum period.[10–12,15] In appropriately counseled women, radiation therapy is possible with fetal doses that fall below the threshold of 5 rad (50 mGy).[28]

Prognosis

Several case series have described prognostic outcome in women diagnosed with breast cancer during pregnancy. Some studies have suggested decreased survival among pregnant women with breast cancer compared with stage-matched controls.[7–9] In contrast, other studies have indicated equal prognosis for pregnancy-associated breast cancer in comparison to nonpregnant women.[5,16,29]

Rodriquez and colleagues[7] published findings from the California Cancer Registry from between 1991 and 1999. In this study, 797 pregnancy-associated breast cancers were compared with 4177 nonpregnant breast cancer controls. After controlling for stage of disease, size of tumor, hormone receptor status, age, race, and type of surgery, survival was reported as worse in pregnancy-associated breast cancer compared with nonpregnant breast cancer controls ($P = .046$).[7] It is unclear if findings are due to delay in diagnosis or less-aggressive therapy due to pregnancy.

In contrast, Beadle and colleagues[29] evaluated 652 women with breast cancer, ages less than or equal to 35 years, who were diagnosed during pregnancy or within the first postpartum year. Women with pregnancy-associated breast cancer had no statistically significant difference in 10-year rates of locoregional recurrence, distant metastasis, or overall survival compared with women who did not have pregnancy-associated breast cancer.[29]

The prognosis of breast cancer in pregnancy seems relate to advanced stages at diagnosis as well as delays in treatment initiation over concern for fetal outcomes. Pregnancy itself does not seem to compromise prognosis. These studies highlight the importance of timely diagnosis and treatment; when women receive timely therapy, there seems no significant difference in outcomes.

Termination

The decision to terminate pregnancy should be individualized. Women should be fully informed of their options and made aware that termination does not improve the outcome of pregnancy-associated breast cancer.[16] Cardonick and colleagues[16] found that survival in those who elected termination was approximately 83% (5 of 6) and, in those with a live born, survival was approximately 85% (81 of 95). There was no significant difference in survival for primary disease if a patient elected termination of pregnancy, had a spontaneous miscarriage, or continued the pregnancy and delivered a live-born infant.[16] Additional factors that should be considered in counseling are patient's willingness to accept a possible risk to the fetus from treatment, overall prognosis, and the ability to care for offspring.[4] The decision to continue or end a pregnancy is a personal one and should be supported by a patient's medical teams.

PRENATAL CARE

A multidisciplinary team should be involved in the care of pregnant women with breast cancer. This team should include an obstetrician, maternal-fetal medicine specialist, medical oncologist, surgical oncologist, geneticist, and neonatologist. Women with breast cancer in pregnancy should be referred for genetic counseling and offered BRCA testing.[10] Pregnant women with breast cancer can be followed per standard prenatal care protocols. At diagnosis, an ultrasound confirming dates is encouraged to provide adequate counseling regarding pregnancy management.[12,15] Additionally, a detailed fetal anatomic evaluation at 20 weeks' gestation is recommended to exclude preexisting fetal anomalies before treatment initiation.[12,15] Pregnancy-related complications should be managed based on the current standard of care.

Once systemic therapy is initiated, fetal monitoring for fetal well-being and general development before each chemotherapy cycle is suggested. The most common outcome associated with chemotherapy is intrauterine growth restriction, and growth scans every 4 weeks, starting at approximately 24 to 28 weeks, are recommended. If there is growth restriction, usual guidelines for monitoring of intrauterine growth restriction should be followed, including biophysical profile with Doppler studies. Chemotherapy during pregnancy should not be given after 35 weeks or within 3 weeks of planned delivery to avoid problems associated with myelosuppression in the mother and fetus, and to avoid drug accumulation in the fetus.[4,10–12] During surgery, the supine position should be avoided after 20 weeks and, once the fetus has reached viability, intraoperative fetal monitoring should take place according to American College of Obstetricians and Gynecologists recommendations.[30]

Timing of delivery should take into account maternal status, need for further therapy, and expected fetal outcome.[4] Iatrogenic preterm delivery should be avoided; however, there may be indications for late preterm delivery (34–36 weeks' gestation) and such cases should be individualized, taking into account maternal and fetal outcomes. Mode of delivery should be determined by usual obstetric indications and delivery should occur in a tertiary center. After delivery, the placenta should be sent for pathology examination.

In the postpartum period, chemotherapy and radiation therapy can be started immediately after a vaginal delivery, and an interval of a week is recommended after an uncomplicated cesarean section.[12] Breastfeeding is contraindicated during treatment with chemotherapy or radiation therapy.[11,12]

SUMMARY

Pregnancy-associated breast cancer poses unique challenges to both mother and fetus. The approach to care of pregnant women with breast cancer should be multidisciplinary and the treatment planned with consideration of the risks to the developing fetus. Mastectomy with anthracycline-based chemotherapy is the most common treatment regimen used. Chemotherapy should be given in the second and third trimesters to minimize risk to the fetus. The reported fetal malformation rate among those exposed to chemotherapy does not seem higher than that reported in the general population, and there do not seem to be any long-term adverse effects among children exposed to chemotherapy. As women delay childbearing, the incidence of pregnancy-associated breast cancer is expected to increase and further research in this field is needed.

REFERENCES

1. Centers for Disease Control and Prevention. Available at: http://www.cdc.gov/cancer/dcpc/data/women.htm. Accessed January 13, 2013.
2. Smith LH, Danielsen B, Allen ME, et al. Cancer associated with obstetric delivery: results of linkage with the California cancer registry. Am J Obstet Gynecol 2003; 189(4):1128–35.
3. Abenhaim HA, Azoulay L, Holcroft CA, et al. Incidence, risk factors, and obstetrical outcomes of women with breast cancer in pregnancy. Breast J 2012;18(6): 564–8.
4. Cohn D, Ramaswamy B, Blum K. Malignancy and pregnancy. In: Creasy R, Iams J, Resnik R, editors. Maternal-fetal medicine principles and practice. 6th edition. Toronto: WB Saunders; 2010. p. 885–904.
5. Ishida T, Yokoe T, Kasmu F, et al. Clinicopathologic characteristics and prognosis of breast cancer patients associated with pregnancy and lactation: Analysis of case-control study in Japan. Jpn J Cancer Res 1992;83:1143–9.
6. Middleton LP, Amin M, Gwyn K, et al. Breast carcinoma in pregnant women: assessment of clinicopathologic and immunohistochemical features. Cancer 2003;98(5):1055–60.
7. Rodriguez AO, Chew H, Cress R, et al. Evidence of poorer survival in pregnancy-associated breast cancer. Obstet Gynecol 2008;112(1):71–8.
8. Ulery M, Carter L, McFarlin BL, et al. Pregnancy-associated breast cancer: significance of early detection. J Midwifery Womens Health 2009;54(5):357–63.

9. Johansson AL, Andersson TM, Hsieh C, et al. Increased mortality in women with breast cancer detected during pregnancy and different periods postpartum. Cancer Epidemiol Biomarkers Prev 2011;20(9):1865–72.

10. Loibl S, von Minckwitz G, Gwyn K, et al. Breast carcinoma during pregnancy. International recommendations from an expert meeting. Cancer 2006;106(2):237–46.

11. Litton JK, Theriault RL. Breast cancer and pregnancy: current concepts in diagnosis and treatment. Oncologist 2010;15(12):1238–47.

12. Amant F, Loibl S, Neven P, et al. Breast cancer in pregnancy. Lancet 2012;379(9815):570–9.

13. Yang WT, Dryden MJ, Gwyn K, et al. Imaging of breast cancer diagnosed and treated with chemotherapy during pregnancy. Radiology 2006;239(1):52–60.

14. Robbins J, Jeffries D, Robidoux M, et al. The accuracy of diagnostic mammography and breast ultrasound during pregnancy and lactation. AJR Am J Roentgenol 2011;196(3):716–22.

15. National Comprehensive Cancer Network. NCCN guidelines version 3.2012 Breast Cancer. Available at: http://www.nccn.org/professionals/physician_gls/pdf/breast.pdf. Accessed January 15, 2013.

16. Cardonick E, Dougherty R, Grana G, et al. Breast cancer during pregnancy: maternal and fetal outcomes. Cancer J 2010;16(1):76–82.

17. Dominici LS, Kuerer HM, Babiera G, et al. Wound complications from surgery in pregnancy-associated breast cancer (PABC). Breast Dis 2010;31(1):1–5.

18. Gentilini O, Cremonesi M, Toesca A, et al. Sentinel lymph node biopsy in pregnant patients with breast cancer. Eur J Nucl Med Mol Imaging 2010;37(1):78–83.

19. Keleher A, Wendt R, Delpassand E, et al. The safety of lymphatic mapping in pregnant breast cancer patients using Tc-99m sulfur colloid. Breast J 2004;10(6):492–5.

20. Hahn KM, Johnson PH, Gordon N, et al. Treatment of pregnant breast cancer patients and outcomes of children exposed to chemotherapy in utero. Cancer 2006;107(6):1219–26.

21. Cardonick E, Bhat A, Gilmandyar D, et al. Maternal and fetal outcomes of taxane chemotherapy in breast and ovarian cancer during pregnancy: case series and review of the literature. Ann Oncol 2012;23(12):3016–23.

22. Mir O, Berveiller P, Goffinet F, et al. Taxanes for breast cancer during pregnancy: a systematic review. Ann Oncol 2010;21(2):425–6.

23. Bonilla L, Ben Aharon I, Vidal L, et al. Dose-dense chemotherapy in nonmetastatic breast cancer: a systematic review and meta-analysis of randomized controlled trials. J Natl Cancer Inst 2010;102(24):1845–54.

24. Cardonick E, Gilmandyar D, Somer RA. Maternal and neonatal outcomes of dose-dense chemotherapy for breast cancer in pregnancy. Obstet Gynecol 2012;120(6):1267–72.

25. Zagouri F, Sergentanis TN, Chrysikos D, et al. Trastuzumab administration during pregnancy: a systematic review and meta-analysis. Breast Cancer Res Treat 2013;137(2):349–57.

26. Isaacs RJ, Hunter W, Clark K. Tamoxifen as systemic treatment of advanced breast cancer during pregnancy—case report and literature review. Gynecol Oncol 2001;80(3):405–8.

27. Pradat P, Robert Gnansia E, Di Tanna GL, et al. First trimester exposure to corticosteroids and oral clefts. Birth Defects Res A Clin Mol Teratol 2003;67(12):968–70.

28. Martin D. Review of radiation therapy in the pregnant cancer patient. Clin Obstet Gynecol 2011;54(4):591–601.

29. Beadle BM, Woodward WA, Middleton LP, et al. The impact of pregnancy on breast cancer outcomes in women ≤35 years. Cancer 2009;115(6):1174–84.
30. American College of Obstetricians and Gynecologists. ACOG Committee Opinion no. 474, February 2011. Nonobstetric surgery during pregnancy. Obstet Gynecol 2011;117:420–1.

Special Considerations in Early-stage Breast Cancer Patients and Survivors

Amelia B. Zelnak, MD, MSc

KEYWORDS

- Breast cancer • Survivorship • Subtypes • Genomic profiling

KEY POINTS

- Genomic profiling has led to the identification of different subtypes of breast cancer, each with a unique gene expression pattern.
- Several assays, such as the 21-gene recurrence score and 70-gene signature, are currently used in clinical practice to assess the molecular profile of a tumor before making recommendations for adjuvant systemic therapy.
- Incorporation of genomic profiling into future clinical trials could lead to improvements in identification of new targets, therapy selection, and improvement in long-term outcomes for breast cancer patients.

INTRODUCTION

More than 200,000 women are expected to be diagnosed with breast cancer in 2013, most of whom will have early-stage disease.[1] As improvements have been made in early detection and treatment, more and more patients have become long-term breast cancer survivors. Many of these patients will have undergone breast surgery, received chemotherapy and radiation therapy, and taken antiestrogen therapy for 5 to 10 years to reduce their risk of developing recurrent disease. Although breast cancer–specific outcomes have improved over time, increased risk of toxicity has also been seen with multimodality therapy.

For many early-stage patients, breast cancer and the resulting survivorship issues are their most significant medical concerns. Long-term follow-up of breast cancer patients has shown that fatigue, sleep disturbances, psychological distress from cancer diagnosis, and menopausal symptoms persisted after they completed their breast

Disclosures: The author has nothing to disclose.
Department of Hematology and Medical Oncology, Winship Cancer Institute, Emory University School of Medicine, 1365 Clifton Road Northeast, Atlanta, GA 30322, USA
E-mail address: amelia.zelnak@emory.edu

Obstet Gynecol Clin N Am 40 (2013) 573–582
http://dx.doi.org/10.1016/j.ogc.2013.05.007

cancer treatment.[2] Patients may also experience lymphedema, neuropathy, osteoporosis, and changes in fertility as a result of their breast cancer treatment.[3] These problems can have significant impact on a patient's quality of life and are frequently discussed by patient and provider during follow-up care.

GUIDELINES FOR FOLLOW-UP OF EARLY-STAGE BREAST CANCER PATIENTS

Current recommendations for follow-up of early-stage breast cancer patients include a visit with a breast cancer provider every 3 to 6 months for the first 3 years, every 6 months in years 4 and 5, and annually thereafter.[4,5] Patients should undergo a clinical breast examination at each visit and be assessed for signs and symptoms of recurrent disease, such as bone pain, chest pain, dyspnea, abdominal pain, or persistent headaches.

Patients who underwent breast-conserving surgery and radiation therapy should have a mammogram of the affected breast performed at least 6 months after completion of radiation. Repeat mammograms are obtained every 6 to 12 months for surveillance of abnormalities. Once stability of mammographic changes is confirmed, patients should then have annual mammograms performed. In asymptomatic patients without any specific evidence of recurrent disease on examination, routine blood work, including tumor markers (carcinoembryonic antigen, CA 15-3, and CA 27.29), complete blood cell count, and chemistry panels, is not routinely recommended. In addition, the routine use of bone scans, CT scans, and positron emission tomography scans is not recommended. Patients who develop symptoms suggestive of recurrent disease should have the appropriate diagnostic tests performed. Regular gynecologic follow-up is recommended for all women. For breast cancer patients who are taking tamoxifen, annual pelvic examination is recommended. Due to the increased risk of endometrial cancer on tamoxifen, all patients should contact their physician immediately if they experience abnormal vaginal bleeding.

ROLE OF ADJUVANT ENDOCRINE THERAPY AND POTENTIAL TOXICITIES

Breast cancer is a heterogeneous disease comprised of different subtypes defined at clinical, pathologic, and molecular levels. In clinical practice, oncologists have recognized for years that the behavior of breast cancers is variable. Assessment of hormone receptor and HER2 status is standard of care at the time of breast cancer diagnosis and currently used to guide adjuvant therapy recommendations. Approximately two-thirds of breast cancers express the estrogen receptor and/or progesterone receptor, and 5 years of adjuvant antiestrogen therapy with either tamoxifen or an aromatase inhibitor (AI) has become standard of care for these based on results from multiple trials.[6] The addition of AIs in the adjuvant setting for postmenopausal women has improved disease-free survival compared with tamoxifen alone. AIs can be used as up-front continuous treatment for 5 years,[7,8] as sequential therapy after 2 to 3 years of tamoxifen[9,10] or as extended adjuvant therapy after 5 years of tamoxifen.[11]

Patients with hormone receptor–positive breast cancer continue to have relapse rates of 1% to 4% per year between 5 and 15 years from diagnosis, and the optimal duration of adjuvant hormonal therapy remains an important clinical question.[12,13] Long-term results of the ATLAS (Adjuvant Tamoxifen: Longer Against Shorter) trial were recently presented, indicating that 10 years of adjuvant tamoxifen resulted in a further reduction in recurrence and mortality compared with 5 years, with continued benefit seen beyond 10 years of therapy.[14] These results are most relevant for premenopausal patients for whom extended adjuvant therapy with an AI is not an alternative option.

Tamoxifen

Tamoxifen is a selective estrogen receptor modulator, which has antiestrogenic effects on some tissues, including the breast, and has partial estrogenic effects elsewhere in the body. This complex mechanism of action results in a side-effect profile with both beneficial and detrimental effects. The most common side effects that patients experience are hot flashes and vaginal complaints (discharge and dryness). Some patients also report weight gain, fatigue, nausea, arthralgias, and irregular menses. Tamoxifen has been shown to improve bone density and may reduce risk of osteoporotic fractures.[15,16] Tamoxifen has been shown to have beneficial effects on the lipid profile, lowering total cholesterol, mainly due to its effect on low-density lipoprotein cholesterol.[17] An increased incidence of deep venous thrombosis and pulmonary embolism has been observed in tamoxifen-treated women.[18]

Tamoxifen has been associated with an increased incidence of endometrial carcinoma in both treatment and prevention of breast cancer due to its proestrogenic effects in the uterus.[18,19] The relative risk of endometrial cancer in the tamoxifen-treated women from the National Surgical Adjuvant Breast and Bowel Project P-1 prevention trial was 2.5. The increased risk was predominantly seen in women over age 50 in whom the relative risk was 4. All the endometrial cancers seen in the tamoxifen-treated women were International Federation of Gynecology and Obstetrics stage I. The tumors were of good prognosis, and none of the women treated with tamoxifen died from endometrial cancer on this trial.

Tamoxifen is metabolized by the cytochrome P450 enzyme, CYP2D6, resulting in the formation of endoxifen. Low to absent CYP2D6 activity due to a common genetic variation has been shown to lower the plasma concentration of endoxifen.[20] Multiple retrospective studies have examined the significance of CYP2D6 activity, levels of endoxifen, and risk of breast cancer recurrence with conflicting results.[21–24] Additional analysis of CYP2D6 phenotype in large, phase 3 randomized trials showed that reduced CYP2D6 activity was not associated with a worse breast cancer outcome among patients taking tamoxifen.[25,26] Based on these results, CYP2D6 testing should not be used in making decisions about whether to prescribe tamoxifen.

Selective serotonin reuptake inhibitor (SSRI) antidepressants have also be shown to inhibit CYP2D6 activity, resulting in lower endoxifen levels.[27] Certain SSRIs, such as paroxetine, fluoxetine, and sertraline, are stronger inhibitors of CYP2D6 activity. Venlafaxine was the weakest CYP2D6 inhibitor among the antidepressants tested. SSRIs are commonly used among early-stage breast cancer patients for management of hot flashes and mood disorders, and the potential interaction with tamoxifen should be considered when making recommendations regarding which SSRI to use, with preference given to weaker inhibitors of CYP2D6 activity.

Aromatase Inhibitors

AIs—anastrozole, letrozole, and exemestane—prevent the peripheral conversion of androstenedione into estrogen, resulting in decreased levels of circulating estrogen.[28,29] AIs are not effective in the management of premenopausal breast cancer patients in whom the ovaries are the main source of estrogen. The main side effects from AIs are hot flashes, musculoskeletal pain, vaginal dryness, and headache. The significant decrease in estrogen levels, however, results in an increased risk of bone loss and resultant osteopenia and osteoporosis.[30] Patients on an AI are recommended to take calcium and vitamin D. They should also have bone density scans performed at baseline and every 1 to 2 years while on an AI. Trials have investigated the role of oral and intravenous bisphosphonate therapy to maintain or improve bone density while on an AI, and they have shown that early bone loss could be prevented.[31] The risks of endometrial cancer, venous thromboembolic disease, vaginal bleeding or discharge, and hot flashes were lower in patients treated with an AI compared with tamoxifen, although the likelihood of musculoskeltal complaints is increased.

Adverse effects on lipid profiles have been suggested, but a clinically significant increase in risk of cardiovascular disease has not been seen in the major studies of AIs. A study evaluated the effect of short-term therapy with 16 weeks of letrozole on plasma lipid profiles. This study found a statistically significant increase in total cholesterol and low-density lipoprotein as well as unfavorable changes in the total cholesterol/high-density lipoprotein and low-density lipoprotein/high-density lipoprotein ratios.[32] All of these changes were reversed within a year of withdrawing AI therapy.[33] Another study evaluated differences in plasma lipid profiles between patients taking letrozole (n = 183) and placebo (n = 164) and found no significant change in plasma lipid profiles of these patients.[34]

MANAGEMENT OF VAGINAL BLEEDING IN PATIENTS ON TAMOXIFEN

All women on tamoxifen should undergo annual pelvic examination. Postmenopausal patients on tamoxifen with vaginal bleeding should be evaluated urgently by a gynecologist. They should be evaluated with transvaginal ultrasound of the endometrium and biopsy if indicated because they are at increased risk of developing endometrial cancer. The evaluation of vaginal bleeding can be challenging in premenopausal and perimenopausal breast cancer patients, among whom abnormal uterine bleeding occurs in more than 50% of patients.[35] Many women have experienced chemotherapy-induced menopause, and resumption of their menstrual cycles could occur up to 2 years after completion of chemotherapy. Vaginal bleeding in this patient population may not be abnormal but should still be evaluated. Up to 23% of premenopausal women taking tamoxifen are diagnosed with endometrial polyps, hyperplasia, or, rarely, cancer; however, this incidence is not significantly different from premenopausal patients who are not taking tamoxifen.[36] Premenopausal women treated with tamoxifen often have irregular menses, making assessment of menstrual cycles more difficult.[37]

Initial evaluation of abnormal vaginal bleeding includes transvaginal ultrasound for endometrial thickness. The likelihood of endometrial cancer increases with endometrial thickness greater than 5 mm in postmenopausal women[38] and over 8 mm to 12 mm in premenopausal patients.[39] Endometrial biopsy should be pursued. If benign, patients should be observed with periodic endometrial ultrasound and biopsy only if indicated based on symptoms. There are currently no data to support routine screening sonography of asymptomatic women on tamoxifen for endometrial cancer.

MANAGEMENT OF ATROPHIC VAGINITIS

Tamoxifen and AIs commonly cause vaginal atrophy, dryness, dyspareunia, and urinary urgency and frequency due to their antiestrogenic effects. The incidence is higher with the AIs compared with tamoxifen.[40] Nonestrogenic treatments with lubricants and vaginal moisturizers are preferred as initial treatment.[41] Long-term safety studies of vaginal estrogens in postmenopausal, breast cancer patients are not available. Studies have shown that systemic absorption of vaginal estrogens does occur; however, the clinical significance of this is unknown.[42] Although systemic estrogens should be avoided in patients with hormone receptor–positive breast cancer, a small retrospective study in breast cancer patients using vaginal estrogens has not shown an adverse effect on long-term outcome.[43] For breast cancer patients with severe atrophic vaginitis for whom nonhormonal agents have not provided symptomatic relief, potential risks and benefits of vaginal estrogens should be carefully considered and discussed before initiating treatment.

MANAGEMENT OF MENOPAUSAL SYMPTOMS

Many patients with early-stage breast cancer experience hot flashes, night sweats, sleep disturbances, and mood irritability after their diagnosis. Postmenopausal patients on hormone replacement therapy at the time of their breast cancer diagnosis are told to discontinue this, leading to the recurrence of menopausal symptoms. Perimenopausal patients may develop normal menopausal symptoms at or near the time of their breast cancer diagnosis. Among premenopausal patients who receive chemotherapy, temporary or permanent ovarian suppression is induced. The likelihood of resuming menstrual cycles after chemotherapy decreases as patients increase in age. Because approximately two-thirds of breast cancer patients are hormone receptor positive, they are treated with antiestrogen therapy in the adjuvant setting, which is known to cause menopausal symptoms.

There are several nonhormonally based treatment options for menopausal symptoms, which may be safely used in breast cancer patients who have severe symptoms that have an impact on their quality of life. SSRIs have been widely tested and used for management of hot flashes in breast cancer patients.[44–46] Patients may also report improvement of sleep disturbances and mood irritability with SSRIs. Most of these studies have compared SSRIs to placebo, and there are few data comparing their efficacy to hormone replacement therapy. SSRIs that are strong inhibitors of CYP2D6, such as paroxetine, fluoxetine, and sertraline, should be avoided, if possible, among women taking tamoxifen. A typical starting dose of venlafaxine for management of hot flashes is 37.5 mg daily, increasing to 75 mg daily if needed.

Gabapentin is currently approved for management of epilepsy and chronic pain but has also been shown to reduce hot flashes in breast cancer patients.[47,48] Unlike SSRIs, gabapentin does not have any potential interactions with tamoxifen. Clonidine has also been shown to have mild to moderate efficacy in treating hot flashes.[49] Menopausal symptoms may improve over time, so it may be reasonable to periodically discontinue medication to reassess severity of symptoms. Patients may also have side effects from the pharmacologic agents used to treat hot flashes. Side effects may also occur when patients abruptly discontinue treatment with SSRIs, and, therefore, these medications should be stopped gradually. Individual breast cancer patients need to consider the severity of their menopausal symptoms and side effects when deciding on how to best manage menopausal symptoms.

PSYCHOLOGICAL ISSUES AMONG EARLY-STAGE BREAST CANCER PATIENTS

Patients often experience symptoms of anxiety and depression when they are initially diagnosed with breast cancer and throughout their treatment course. A study of more than 700 women diagnosed with breast cancer has shown that they are more likely to have anxiety and depression compared with the general population. Anxiety was more common than depression among patients with early-stage breast cancer, and symptoms persisted beyond the time of initial diagnosis.[50] Earlier studies have shown that the percentage of breast cancer patients with symptoms of anxiety was highest around the time of surgery, and was slightly lower 12 months later.[51] Fears of developing recurrent breast cancer do not always dissipate over time. Patients should be assessed for depression and anxiety during their routine follow-up visits. Initiation of an antidepressant is often indicated along with referral for counseling or psycho-therapy. Cancer support groups may also provide additional support for patients.

Fatigue is one of the most common and difficult to manage symptoms in long-term cancer survivors. All aspects of multimodality therapy for early-stage breast cancer, surgery, chemotherapy, radiation therapy, and hormonal therapy have been associ-ated with increased fatigue. Cancer-related fatigue often persists well beyond the time of initial diagnosis.[52,53] Ongoing research has focused on the role of inflammatory signaling as a possible explanation for persistent fatigue, depressive symptoms, and sleep disturbances among breast cancer survivors.[54] Cancer-related fatigue can have significant impact on quality of life. Initial assessment should be focused on treatable contributing factors, such as anemia, side effects from therapy, nutrition, pain, and comorbid conditions.[55] Physical activity has been shown to improve cancer-related fatigue both during and after breast cancer therapy.[56,57] Psychosocial interventions, such as cognitive-behavioral therapy, counseling, and behavioral therapy, also have been associated with small to moderate improvements in cancer-related fatigue.[58]

Patients may also report problems with cognitive function during and after comple-tion of breast cancer therapy. Earlier studies comparing neuropsychologic status of breast cancer patients who received chemotherapy with those who did not show increased cognitive impairment among women who received chemotherapy.[59] Inter-pretation of these studies can be challenging because many did not have baseline assessment of cognitive function before receiving breast cancer therapy. Other studies have shown only subtle differences in cognitive functioning after chemo-therapy for breast cancer.[60,61] Subsequent studies have shown that symptoms of cognitive impairment were most commonly related to attention, learning, and cogni-tive speed.[62,63] There may also be overlap of symptoms in patients who experience cancer-related fatigue, anxiety or depression, and cognitive impairment.

SUMMARY

As outcomes for early-stage breast cancer patients have improved, more patients have become long-term breast cancer survivors. In addition to routine evaluation for recurrent disease with breast imaging and clinical examination, clinicians should care-fully assess for potential side effects of therapy. Menopausal symptoms, mood irrita-bility, and anxiety and depression may improve with antidepressants, such as SSRIs. Counseling and support groups may play a key role, however, in helping breast cancer patients improve their quality of life. Additional research into the etiology of cancer-related fatigue may provide new insight into management of early-stage breast cancer patients.

REFERENCES

1. American Cancer Society. Cancer facts & figures 2013. Atlanta (GA): American Cancer Society; 2013.
2. Dow KH, Ferrell BR, Leigh S, et al. An evaluation of the quality of life among long-term survivors of breast cancer. Breast Cancer Res Treat 1996;39(3): 261–73.
3. Ganz PA, Hahn EE. Implementing a survivorship care plan for patients with breast cancer. J Clin Oncol 2008;26(5):759–67.
4. Zhu Q, Jin L, Casero RA, et al. Role of ornithine decarboxylase in regulation of estrogen receptor alpha expression and growth in human breast cancer cells. Breast Cancer Res Treat 2012;136(1):57–66.

5. Khatcheressian JL, Hurley P, Bantug E, et al. Breast cancer follow-up and management after primary treatment: American Society of Clinical Oncology clinical practice guideline update. J Clin Oncol 2013;31(7):961–5.
6. Davies C, Godwin J, Gray R, et al. Relevance of breast cancer hormone receptors and other factors to the efficacy of adjuvant tamoxifen: patient-level meta-analysis of randomised trials. Lancet 2011;378(9793):771–84.
7. Cuzick J, Sestak I, Baum M, et al. Effect of anastrozole and tamoxifen as adjuvant treatment for early-stage breast cancer: 10-year analysis of the ATAC trial. Lancet Oncol 2010;11(12):1135–41.
8. Regan MM, Neven P, Giobbie-Hurder A, et al. Assessment of letrozole and tamoxifen alone and in sequence for postmenopausal women with steroid hormone receptor-positive breast cancer: the BIG 1-98 randomised clinical trial at 8.1 years median follow-up. Lancet Oncol 2011;12(12):1101–8.
9. Dubsky PC, Jakesz R, Mlineritsch B, et al. Tamoxifen and anastrozole as a sequencing strategy: a randomized controlled trial in postmenopausal patients with endocrine-responsive early breast cancer from the Austrian Breast and Colorectal Cancer Study Group. J Clin Oncol 2012;30(7):722–8.
10. Bliss JM, Kilburn LS, Coleman RE, et al. Disease-related outcomes with long-term follow-up: an updated analysis of the intergroup exemestane study. J Clin Oncol 2012;30(7):709–17.
11. Jin H, Tu D, Zhao N, et al. Longer-term outcomes of letrozole versus placebo after 5 years of tamoxifen in the NCIC CTG MA.17 trial: analyses adjusting for treatment crossover. J Clin Oncol 2012;30(7):718–21.
12. Group EBCTC. Tamoxifen for early breast cancer cochrane database of systematic reviews: reviews 2001 issue 1. Chichester (United Kingdom): John Wiley & Sons, Ltd; 2001 (Issue 1).
13. Saphner T, Tormey DC, Gray R. Annual hazard rates of recurrence for breast cancer after primary therapy. J Clin Oncol 1996;14(10):2738–46.
14. Davies C, Pan H, Godwin J, et al. Long-term effects of continuing adjuvant tamoxifen to 10 years versus stopping at 5 years after diagnosis of oestrogen receptor-positive breast cancer: ATLAS, a randomised trial. Lancet 2012; 381(9869):805–16.
15. Love RR, Mazess RB, Barden HS, et al. Effects of tamoxifen on bone mineral density in postmenopausal women with breast cancer. N Engl J Med 1992; 326(13):852–6.
16. Kristensen B, Ejlertsen B, Dalgaard P, et al. Tamoxifen and bone metabolism in postmenopausal low-risk breast cancer patients: a randomized study. J Clin Oncol 1994;12(5):992–7.
17. Bruning PF, Bonfrer JM, Hart AA, et al. Tamoxifen, serum lipoproteins and cardiovascular risk. Br J Cancer 1988;58(4):497–9.
18. Fisher B, Costantino JP, Wickerham DL, et al. Tamoxifen for prevention of breast cancer: report of the National Surgical Adjuvant Breast and Bowel Project P-1 Study. J Natl Cancer Inst 1998;90(18):1371–88.
19. Tamoxifen for early breast cancer: an overview of the randomised trials. Early Breast Cancer Trialists' Collaborative Group. Lancet 1998;351(9114):1451–67.
20. Stearns V, Johnson MD, Rae JM, et al. Active tamoxifen metabolite plasma concentrations after coadministration of tamoxifen and the selective serotonin reuptake inhibitor paroxetine. J Natl Cancer Inst 2003;95(23):1758–64.
21. Goetz MP, Rae JM, Suman VJ, et al. Pharmacogenetics of tamoxifen biotransformation is associated with clinical outcomes of efficacy and hot flashes. J Clin Oncol 2005;23(36):9312–8.

22. Nowell SA, Ahn J, Rae JM, et al. Association of genetic variation in tamoxifen-metabolizing enzymes with overall survival and recurrence of disease in breast cancer patients. Breast Cancer Res Treat 2005;91(3):249–58.

23. Wegman PP, Wingren S. CYP2D6 variants and the prediction of tamoxifen response in randomized patients: author response. Breast Cancer Res 2005; 7(6):E7.

24. Schroth W, Antoniadou L, Fritz P, et al. Breast cancer treatment outcome with adjuvant tamoxifen relative to patient CYP2D6 and CYP2C19 genotypes. J Clin Oncol 2007;25(33):5187–93.

25. Regan MM, Leyland-Jones B, Bouzyk M, et al. CYP2D6 genotype and tamoxifen response in postmenopausal women with endocrine-responsive breast cancer: the breast international group 1-98 trial. J Natl Cancer Inst 2012;104(6):441–51.

26. Rae JM, Drury S, Hayes DF, et al. CYP2D6 and UGT2B7 genotype and risk of recurrence in tamoxifen-treated breast cancer patients. J Natl Cancer Inst 2012;104(6):452–60.

27. Jin Y, Desta Z, Stearns V, et al. CYP2D6 genotype, antidepressant use, and tamoxifen metabolism during adjuvant breast cancer treatment. J Natl Cancer Inst 2005;97(1):30–9.

28. Judd HL, Judd GE, Lucas WE, et al. Endocrine function of the postmenopausal ovary: concentration of androgens and estrogens in ovarian and peripheral vein blood. J Clin Endocrinol Metab 1974;39(6):1020–4.

29. Richards JS, Hickey GJ, Chen SA, et al. Hormonal regulation of estradiol biosynthesis, aromatase activity, and aromatase mRNA in rat ovarian follicles and corpora lutea. Steroids 1987;50(4–6):393–409.

30. Howell A, Cuzick J, Baum M, et al. Results of the ATAC (Arimidex, Tamoxifen, Alone or in Combination) trial after completion of 5 years' adjuvant treatment for breast cancer. Lancet 2005;365(9453):60–2.

31. Brufsky A, Harker WG, Beck JT, et al. Zoledronic acid inhibits adjuvant letrozole-induced bone loss in postmenopausal women with early breast cancer. J Clin Oncol 2007;25(7):829–36.

32. Elisaf MS, Bairaktari ET, Nicolaides C, et al. Effect of letrozole on the lipid profile in postmenopausal women with breast cancer. Eur J Cancer 2001;37(12): 1510–3.

33. Geisler J, Lonning PE, Krag LE, et al. Changes in bone and lipid metabolism in postmenopausal women with early breast cancer after terminating 2-year treatment with exemestane: a randomised, placebo-controlled study. Eur J Cancer 2006;42(17):2968–75.

34. Wasan KM, Goss PE, Pritchard PH, et al. The influence of letrozole on serum lipid concentrations in postmenopausal women with primary breast cancer who have completed 5 years of adjuvant tamoxifen (NCIC CTG MA.17L). Ann Oncol 2005;16(5):707–15.

35. Buijs C, Willemse PH, de Vries EG, et al. Effect of tamoxifen on the endometrium and the menstrual cycle of premenopausal breast cancer patients. Int J Gynecol Cancer 2009;19(4):677–81.

36. Cheng WF, Lin HH, Torng PL, et al. Comparison of endometrial changes among symptomatic tamoxifen-treated and nontreated premenopausal and postmenopausal breast cancer patients. Gynecol Oncol 1997;66(2):233–7.

37. Runowicz CD, Costantino JP, Wickerham DL, et al. Gynecologic conditions in participants in the NSABP breast cancer prevention study of tamoxifen and raloxifene (STAR). Am J Obstet Gynecol 2011;205(6):535.e1–5.

38. Karlsson B, Granberg S, Wikland M, et al. Transvaginal ultrasonography of the endometrium in women with postmenopausal bleeding–a Nordic multicenter study. Am J Obstet Gynecol 1995;172(5):1488–94.
39. Ozdemir S, Celik C, Gezginc K, et al. Evaluation of endometrial thickness with transvaginal ultrasonography and histopathology in premenopausal women with abnormal vaginal bleeding. Arch Gynecol Obstet 2010;282(4):395–9.
40. Fallowfield L, Cella D, Cuzick J, et al. Quality of life of postmenopausal women in the Arimidex, Tamoxifen, Alone or in Combination (ATAC) Adjuvant Breast Cancer Trial. J Clin Oncol 2004;22(21):4261–71.
41. Ganz PA. Breast cancer, menopause, and long-term survivorship: critical issues for the 21st century. Am J Med 2005;118(Suppl 12B):136–41.
42. Labrie F, Cusan L, Gomez JL, et al. Effect of one-week treatment with vaginal estrogen preparations on serum estrogen levels in postmenopausal women. Menopause 2009;16(1):30–6.
43. Dew JE, Wren BG, Eden JA. A cohort study of topical vaginal estrogen therapy in women previously treated for breast cancer. Climacteric 2003;6(1):45–52.
44. Stearns V. Clinical update: new treatments for hot flushes. Lancet 2007; 369(9579):2062–4.
45. Speroff L, Gass M, Constantine G, et al. Efficacy and tolerability of desvenlafaxine succinate treatment for menopausal vasomotor symptoms: a randomized controlled trial. Obstet Gynecol 2008;111(1):77–87.
46. Freeman EW, Guthrie KA, Caan B, et al. Efficacy of escitalopram for hot flashes in healthy menopausal women: a randomized controlled trial. JAMA 2011; 305(3):267–74.
47. Loprinzi CL, Kugler JW, Barton DL, et al. Phase III trial of gabapentin alone or in conjunction with an antidepressant in the management of hot flashes in women who have inadequate control with an antidepressant alone: NCCTG N03C5. J Clin Oncol 2007;25(3):308–12.
48. Pandya KJ, Morrow GR, Roscoe JA, et al. Gabapentin for hot flashes in 420 women with breast cancer: a randomised double-blind placebo-controlled trial. Lancet 2005;366(9488):818–24.
49. Nelson HD, Vesco KK, Haney E, et al. Nonhormonal therapies for menopausal hot flashes: systematic review and meta-analysis. JAMA 2006;295(17): 2057–71.
50. Osborne RH, Elsworth GR, Hopper JL. Age-specific norms and determinants of anxiety and depression in 731 women with breast cancer recruited through a population-based cancer registry. Eur J Cancer 2003;39(6):755–62.
51. Fallowfield LJ, Hall A, Maguire GP, et al. Psychological outcomes of different treatment policies in women with early breast cancer outside a clinical trial. BMJ 1990;301(6752):575–80.
52. Ganz PA, Bower JE. Cancer related fatigue: a focus on breast cancer and Hodgkin's disease survivors. Acta Oncol 2007;46(4):474–9.
53. Bower JE, Ganz PA, Desmond KA, et al. Fatigue in breast cancer survivors: occurrence, correlates, and impact on quality of life. J Clin Oncol 2000;18(4): 743–53.
54. Bower JE, Ganz PA, Irwin MR, et al. Inflammation and behavioral symptoms after breast cancer treatment: do fatigue, depression, and sleep disturbance share a common underlying mechanism? J Clin Oncol 2011;29(26):3517–22.
55. Berger AM, Gerber LH, Mayer DK. Cancer-related fatigue: implications for breast cancer survivors. Cancer 2012;118(Suppl 8):2261–9.

56. McNeely ML, Campbell KL, Rowe BH, et al. Effects of exercise on breast cancer patients and survivors: a systematic review and meta-analysis. CMAJ 2006; 175(1):34–41.
57. Markes M, Brockow T, Resch KL. Exercise for women receiving adjuvant therapy for breast cancer. Cochrane Database Syst Rev 2006;(4):CD005001.
58. Kangas M, Bovbjerg DH, Montgomery GH. Cancer-related fatigue: a systematic and meta-analytic review of non-pharmacological therapies for cancer patients. Psychol Bull 2008;134(5):700–41.
59. van Dam FS, Schagen SB, Muller MJ, et al. Impairment of cognitive function in women receiving adjuvant treatment for high-risk breast cancer: high-dose versus standard-dose chemotherapy. J Natl Cancer Inst 1998;90(3):210–8.
60. Jim HS, Donovan KA, Small BJ, et al. Cognitive functioning in breast cancer survivors: a controlled comparison. Cancer 2009;115(8):1776–83.
61. Donovan KA, Small BJ, Andrykowski MA, et al. Cognitive functioning after adjuvant chemotherapy and/or radiotherapy for early-stage breast carcinoma. Cancer 2005;104(11):2499–507.
62. Wefel JS, Lenzi R, Theriault R, et al. 'Chemobrain' in breast carcinoma? A prologue. Cancer 2004;101(3):466–75.
63. Wefel JS, Lenzi R, Theriault RL, et al. The cognitive sequelae of standard-dose adjuvant chemotherapy in women with breast carcinoma: results of a prospective, randomized, longitudinal trial. Cancer 2004;100(11):2292–9.

Medicolegal Considerations in Breast Health

The Benefits of Collaboration Between OB/GYNs and Radiologists

Lisa S. Mitchell, MBA[a],*, Lisa Atkinson, RTR(M), BS[b],
Catherine Hagan-Aylor, BA, BSN, MSN, CBCN[b], Beverly H. Binner, JD[c],
Emily Gannon, BS[a], Patrice M. Weiss, MD[d], Eileen Kenny, MD[b]

KEYWORDS

- Medical malpractice • Medicolegal • Delayed diagnosis
- Clinical Breast Exam (CBE) • Shared decision-making • Mammography facility
- Mammography standards

KEY POINTS

- Radiologists and obstetrician/gynecologists collaborating together for evidence-based clinical practice to diagnose, care for, and treat women with breast disease offers benefit to their patients in improved outcomes.
- Delayed diagnosis of breast cancer is a leading source of litigation for the obstetrician/gynecologist and the radiologist.
- Developing shared checklists between the radiologists and the obstetrician/gynecologist may result in improved communication and decreased litigation.
- Patient's presenting with breast complaints should generally be scheduled for a diagnostic mammogram (likely including ultrasound imaging) rather than a screening procedure.
- Practitioners should choose radiology facilities for referral based on quality metrics including performance of at least 480 screening mammograms/years, positive predictive value of screen; minimal, incident, and prevalent cancers found.

INTRODUCTION

In a recent article in *Radiology*, Whang and colleagues[1] found with 95% confidence that the most "common general cause" of malpractice suits against radiologists stems from error in diagnosis—and breast cancer is the most frequently missed diagnosis in

Disclosures: The authors have nothing to disclose.
[a] Department of Radiology, Carilion Clinic, Roanoke, VA 24018, USA; [b] Carilion Clinic Breast Care Center, Department of Radiology, Carilion Clinic, Roanoke, VA 24018, USA; [c] Carilion Clinic Legal Department, Carilion Clinic, Roanoke, VA 24018, USA; [d] Department of Obstetrics/Gynecology, Carilion Clinic, Roanoke, VA 24018, USA
* Corresponding author.
E-mail address: lxmitchell@carilionclinic.org

Obstet Gynecol Clin N Am 40 (2013) 583–597
http://dx.doi.org/10.1016/j.ogc.2013.05.005
0889-8545/13/$ – see front matter © 2013 Elsevier Inc. All rights reserved.

the category. Missed breast cancer diagnoses raise both medical and legal concerns for radiologists, and the issue is an increasing legal concern for their practices, even more so than medical concerns. In 1995, a 20-year review of trends in malpractice claims against radiologists demonstrated missed diagnoses as the leading cause of action, increasing from 34% to 47% over the 20 years, with the greatest increase attributed to the missed breast cancer diagnoses.[2]

Obstetrician/gynecologists (OB/Gyns) face an even more hostile medicolegal environment, as described in 2 recent reports issued by the American Congress of Gynecologists and Obstetricians (ACOG). So much is this the case that James T. Breeden, MD, president of ACOG, leader in the field of OB/Gyn practice, in 2012 categorized the ongoing and unchanged nature of today's medicolegal environment for OB/Gyns as a "crisis."[3] Specifically, ACOG's 2012 professional liability assessment revealed "no overall improvement of the medicolegal environment for OB/Gyns."[3] Even more alarming is that 63% of OB/Gyns indicated they changed their practices by reducing surgical procedures and high-risk patients "due to the risk or fear of being sued."[3] This fear is well-founded in light of even more sobering statistics that 90% of OB/Gyns will be sued at least once during their career, although 53% of closed claims for 2006 to 2008 were dropped, dismissed, or settled.[4] One-third of these claims involved gynecologic care. "Delayed or failure to diagnose" accounted for 22% of the gynecologic claims, second only to patient injury; of the "delay in or failure to diagnose," cancer was the major allegation of these cancer-related claims, with the most frequently cited being breast cancer. Moreover, OB/Gyns continue to have more paid claims than any of the other medical specialties. This challenging environment for OB/Gyns and the high risk of litigation associated with missed diagnosis of breast cancer is an opportunity for radiologists and OB/Gyns to partner in addressing the best safeguards and preparedness for potential lawsuits.

Radiologists and OB/Gyns collaborating for evidence-based clinical practice to diagnose, care for, and treat women with breast disease also offers benefit to their patients in improved outcomes. A survey report in the New England Journal of Medicine focused on following standard practices as a "key element of quality."[5] Two standard practices ranked as problematic due to being underused were appropriate follow-up of a palpable mass and the choice of surgical treatments for stage I or II cancers.[5] Navigating patients through complex decision-making in breast cancer diagnosis requires a team that coordinates care.[6] Furthermore, for patients diagnosed with localized or regional (spread to nearby lymph nodes) breast cancer, 5-year survival rates are highest at 99% and 84%, respectively,[7] compelling a coordinated approach to standardized, evidence-based practice created by OB/Gyns and radiologists.

EVIDENCE-BASED MEDICINE TRANSCENDS DEFENSIVE MEDICINE

As opposed to taking a defensive medicine posture in limiting potential risk for a missed breast cancer diagnosis, a better strategy would be the practice of evidence-based medicine in striving for the best clinical outcomes for women. A defensive medicine approach alone promotes overutilization of diagnostic tests to protect against litigation. On the other hand, standardized processes, such as evidence-based practice and collaboration among physicians, lead to higher quality outcomes for patients. The evidence-based approach is supported in recent literature for legal considerations. Identified in the 2010 Affordable Care Act, the evidence-based approach includes the use of qualified information technology systems and adherence to clinical practice guidelines that do not promote defensive medicine.[8] Furthermore, in keeping with evidence-based practice, development of protocols and checklists is shown to improve outcomes, and their use is strongly encouraged among OB/Gyns to increase quality, collaboration, and interdisciplinary care.[9] Taking this approach in breast care for OB/Gyn patients and in partnership with radiologists produces standardization in communication. To develop a common checklist with radiology and OB-Gyn evidence-based practices, categorizing patient access scenarios and clinical processes provides sharper focus.

ORGANIZE PATIENT FLOW FOR PROTOCOL DEVELOPMENT

OB/Gyns and radiologists should consider the following access scenarios for their patients seeking breast care. First, patients should be categorized as symptomatic of breast problems or asymptomatic of breast problems. Furthermore, for the symptomatic breast patient (SBP), breast problems are either self-identified or clinically palpated in the OB/Gyn office via the clinical breast examination (CBE). The SBP will seek care for her self-identified breast symptoms in 3 ways: (1) seeking clinical evaluation with her health care practitioner; (2) seeking a mammogram with the local breast center mammography location; or (3) watchful waiting, postponing care due to barriers (eg, financial concerns, minimizing the breast symptom due to fear of having breast cancer or fear of the impending examination itself) (**Fig. 1**).

The asymptomatic breast patient (ABP) seeks assessment for breast care by the same 3 avenues: (1) seeking annual examination with her health care practitioner; (2) seeking a screening mammogram with the local breast center screening mammography location; or (3) watchful waiting, postponing choices (1) and (2) because of barriers. Both practices have the opportunity to share checklists and protocols (especially when practices are at differing locations) for handling SBP and ABP. In sharing and committing to shared checklists, OB/Gyns assure adherence to evidence-based standards. Whether the patient is an SBP or ABP, presenting in either the OB/Gyn office or the local screening mammography location is the first access point where a woman's breast cancer diagnosis may be missed (**Fig. 2**).

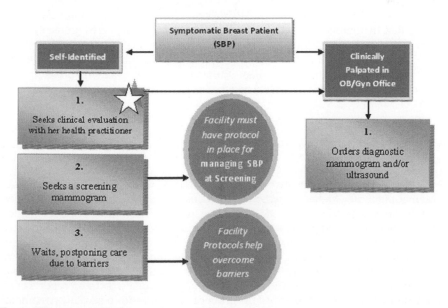

Fig. 1. SBP access scenario.

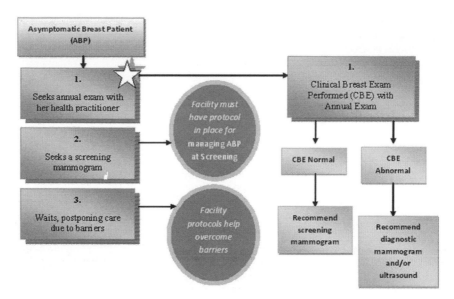

Fig. 2. ABP access scenario.

SBP: A SHARED APPROACH BY THE OB/GYN AND RADIOLOGIST

Clinical management of the SBP with self-reported breast symptoms presenting in the OB/Gyn office setting or in the radiology breast screening site requires a rigorous clinical protocol to assure optimal imaging evaluation. This scenario is a "watershed" moment to assure the best safeguards are in place for the best clinical evaluation. Because a woman may have experienced a CBE or mammogram that is normal and then detects something herself, OB/Gyns and radiologists must assure that both specialties follow a clinical standard of care to manage their patient's understanding that mammograms may miss 15% of breast cancer cases (possibly more missed cases in women with dense breasts).[10] The American College of Radiology (ACR) Practice Guideline for the Performance of Screening and Diagnostic Mammography states that for self-reported breast symptom, other than bilateral breast pain, a facility must have either a "process by which she is converted into a diagnostic case" (**Box 1**) or "there should be some means to have her mammogram brought to the attention of the reading radiologist to avoid delay in reporting" (**Box 2**).[11]

ACR PRACTICE GUIDELINE: TWO OPTIONS FOR SBP WITH SELF-REPORTED SYMPTOM(S)

OB/Gyns should collaborate with the screening facility to which they refer patients, assuring that the facility has either option 1: a process to convert their patient-identified symptomatic women to a diagnostic evaluation; or option 2: rigorous documentation and safeguards to alert reading radiologists to any patient-reported symptoms to avoid any delay in reporting. OB/Gyns should use either option 1 or 2 and confirm documentation in 2 ways from the referral screening facility: (1) through a documented protocol of management of SBP with self-identified breast symptom; and (2) through specific documentation of the self-reported patients in the radiologist's dictated reports back to the OB/Gyn practice—especially if the practice opts to perform screening mammogram, instead of converting to diagnostic mammogram, with option 2. If the screening mammography facility's process is to call OB/Gyn office for an order, which is required by the Centers for Medicare and Medicaid Services (CMS), then the Ob/Gyn office must have a process in place to agree and issue the order for converting to diagnostic evaluation. Recommended processes are shown in **Boxes 1** and **2**.

Physician Practice Question 1

Q: *What if your screening mammography facility calls for an order to convert a patient to diagnostic mammogram and you have not seen the patient in the past year or more?*

A: *Write the order for diagnostic evaluation[a] and schedule a follow-up visit with the patient.*

[a] *Diagnostic evaluation typically includes bilateral diagnostic mammogram and ultrasound.*

Although the ACR Guideline offers the 2 options described above, additional options could include identification of clinical symptoms found in the literature to be most indicative of breast cancer,[12] then converting those women to diagnostic; and refining new clinical symptoms to the following: breast lump, bloody or clear nipple discharge, inverted nipple or skin retraction (unilateral), rash or scaling (nipple/areolar), and swelling.[12] Other patient-reported symptoms are sent directly to the radiologist to avoid delay in interpretation. This additional option offers a refinement to patient-reported breast symptoms converted to diagnostic, compared to those noted directly to radiologists as they interpret screening mammograms. Both the OB/Gyn office and the screening mammography referral location should agree on the clinical symptoms to prompt conversion to diagnostic or notification of the radiologist to expedite interpretation.

Physician Practice Question 2

Q: *What if your screening mammography facility calls for an order to convert a patient to diagnostic mammogram and you performed recent CBE on the patient that was negative?*

A: *Write the order for diagnostic evaluation and schedule a follow-up visit with the patient.*

The Centers for Medicare and Medicaid Services does offer limited reference in the ability for radiologists to convert a woman's order from screening to diagnostic, based on self-reported symptom, independent of the referring OB/Gyn placing the order.[13] Narrow interpretations of this reference result in radiologists not converting existing screening orders to diagnostic. Furthermore, radiologists are more apt not to change an order as a standard, particularly when an OB/Gyn questions changing an order, based on his or her prior CBE of the patient over self-reported symptom.[14] The scenario of an OB/Gyn being unwilling to change a screening mammography order based on recent CBE, when the same patient presents to screening site identifying self-reported breast symptom indicative of breast cancer, is untenable. Only together can OB/Gyns and radiologists communicate patient-reported symptoms and resolve how they manage patients in a collaborative approach to avoid this dilemma. CMS requires that "Radiologic services must be provided only on the order of practitioners with clinical privileges or, consistent with state law, of other practitioners authorized by the medical staff and the governing body to order services."[13] Based on this definition and interpretation, radiologists could convert a screening mammogram for a woman with self-reported symptom to a diagnostic mammogram. Of the limited exceptions, Duszak and Berlin report that some radiology practices are comfortable converting the screening to diagnostic, because this would meet 1 of the 3 exceptions cited by CMS, known as the "clear error" exception.[14]

SBP–OB-GYN PALPATES FINDING DURING CBE

The ideal scenario is for an SBP to seek care for breast problems from her OB/Gyn and thus give the OB/Gyn the opportunity to palpate the breast clinically and examine for changes. Despite the fact that recent literature has debated whether the performance of patient-administered self-breast examination and CBE improves mortality, the importance of conducting CBE and listening to a woman who indicates symptoms and changes in her breasts is paramount to evidence-based care and quality outcome. A recent review indicates CBE does not favorably impact mortality; yet the same analysis detracting against self-breast examination and CBE based on no mortality impact acknowledges the clinical benefit of noting and addressing changes in the breasts that indicate breast cancer.[15] For OB/Gyns, the CBE represents a critical intersection in care to assure breast cancer is not missed.[15] In addition, evaluation of the breast before interventional procedures, including biopsy, is helpful in after procedure evaluation, preventing the scenario of not knowing whether a current lump was present before the procedure (possible hematoma formation) or whether the lump is changing or quickly increasing in size.

CBE, BREAST HEALTH, AND FAMILY HISTORY CHECKLIST

Whether the OB/Gyn palpates clinical findings for his or her patients who present with self-identified symptoms or during the well-woman check-up, standardized communication about the finding, with an order for diagnostic mammogram and/ or breast ultrasound, is needed. A CBE Results Documentation form can be created by the OB/Gyn practice for standardizing quality documentation among physicians and advanced practice clinicians. There are several examples of CBE Results Documentation and Breast Evaluation forms available for reference by physicians. The California Department of Public Health, Cancer Detection Section Breast Expert Workgroup offers one example.[12] A CBE documentation form should describe[12]:

1. Patient-reported concerns: checklist documentation of patient description of breast changes such as:
   a. Lump
   b. Nipple discharge
   c. Thickening
   d. Skin changes
   e. Left/right breast location
2. CBE findings: checklist documentation of the following:
   a. Symmetry
   b. Skin edema
   c. Tenderness
   d. Mass (shape, margins, size, texture, mobility)
   e. Lymph nodes (axillary, clavicular, and whether enlarged, fixed, or mobile)
   f. Left/right breast location
   g. Nodularity
   h. Nipple change
   i. Nipple discharge
3. Overall breast diagram with markings denoting clinical findings (**Fig. 3**).

In addition to the CBE documentation, the form should address the patient's hereditary breast cancer risk based on family history and overall breast treatment history. Furthermore, a case management or referral section to address the next steps for ordering imaging follow-up is shown, including diagnostic evaluation and/or ultrasound only, based on patient age.[12]

WELL-WOMAN VISIT: ELEMENTS OF COMPREHENSIVE BREAST CARE

In ACOG's Committee Opinion for Gynecological Practices, CBE is identified as a "core element" of the well-woman visit. In addition, the opinion mirrors the American Cancer Society and National Comprehensive Cancer Network (NCCN) guidelines for screening CBE in the asymptomatic woman:

A. For women age 20–39, every 1 to 3 years
B. For women age 40 and older, annually
C. Teaching breast self-awareness
D. Assessing a woman's personal and family history for risk factors identified for increased risk of breast disease.[16]

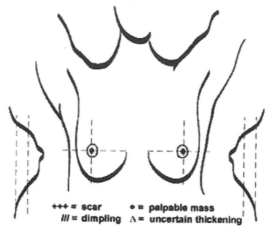

Fig. 3. CBE breast diagram. (*From* California Department of Public Health Cancer Detection Section, Breast Expert Workgroup. Breast Cancer Diagnostic Algorithms for Primary Care Providers. 2011. Available at: http://qap.sdsu.edu/resources/tools/pdf/docform.pdf. Accessed on January 14, 2013.)

Furthermore, these guidelines are endorsed in the Agency for Healthcare Research and Quality (AHRQ) National Guidelines Clearinghouse (NGC) with a "consensus and expert opinion."[17] The AHRQ-NGC also expands on these guidelines and supports

E. Annual screening mammography for women age 40 and older
F. Educating women on the value of screening, including its predictive value, potential for false positives, and further imaging involved (eg, ultrasound) and evaluating women for high risk
    a. For those who test positive for gene mutations, BRCA1 and BRCA2, recommend increased surveillance and discussions regarding how to reduce risk
    b. With women whose lifetime risk of breast cancer is estimated at 20% or greater, based on existing family history models (further discussed in the article by Green elsewhere in this issue), offer increased screening surveillance, which may include magnetic resonance imaging
G. Magnetic resonance imaging is an imaging modality not recommended for screening of average-risk women.

Incorporating elements A–G into the well-woman visit is recommended by authors of this article and addresses a comprehensive approach to breast care. The authors also recommend combining breast awareness education with teaching women that evidence-based literature shows screening mammography in performance and as a tool for early detection is not perfect. Mammography statistics include reported predictive value, false-positives, mammography sensitivity (reported as 84.1% nationally), and mammography specificity (reported as 90.4% nationally).[18] Establishing open communication with women about breast health and the true value of screening can be coordinated between the OB/Gyn practice and the radiologist breast imaging facility. Practices should share current literature about breast health education and the value of screening among physicians and patients. Furthermore, developing a coordinated approach to education, high-risk evaluation, and screening recommendations strengthens evidence-based practices for both specialties while standardizing care.

PATIENT PERSPECTIVE: NAVIGATING INFORMATION IS DIFFICULT

OB/Gyns are well positioned to help their newly diagnosed patients with breast cancer navigate confusion created by a bombardment of information from social media and the Internet. They can provide known accurate clinical information and recommended web sites, which they have researched to meet evidence-based practice recommendations. The patient's now fairly pervasive use of the Internet and social media to research information meticulously about her new cancer diagnosis should be integrated into the OB/Gyn patient's plan of care when she is diagnosed. Access to medical knowledge through social media and the Internet is changing the methods by which patients gain knowledge about health and illness; patients routinely use these tools for probing facts about their initial diagnosis, possible treatment, and follow-up.[19] According to Dr Rita Charon, "It's (social media) a massive revolution. It altogether shifts what goes on when a patient comes in with pages of downloaded stuff and half the time the doctor looking at it has never seen it before. There are a whole new set of emotions present."[20]

Physician Practice Question 3

Q: *Why develop a coordinated approach to breast health education and screening recommendations?*

A: *OB/Gyns are uniquely positioned to navigate patients to accurate, evidence-based information.*

The use of e-mail in communication with patients is also being incorporated into practice settings nationally. The prospective areas for medical liability lie in "confidentiality, privacy, and security," according to the Canadian Medical Protective Association.[21] Although there are advantages and disadvantages of e-mail communication with the patient, summarized in **Boxes 3** and **4**, the OB/Gyn should weigh the risks and benefits of e-mail communication carefully and strategically plan timeliness of responses and clarity of communication as well as consider an informed consent process.[22]

If a physician offers the opportunity for a patient to communicate via e-mail, then the physician and patient should have a clear conversation regarding timeliness of responses and the use of informed consent as to what can be discussed and agreed on. This conversation will avoid circumstances such as unsolicited e-mails. According

---

Box 3
Advantages of e-mail communication

- Ease of use
- Accessible at multiple locations
- Avoid "telephone tag"
- Generates written documentation (self-documentation)
- Reimbursed by some payers
- May improve office efficiency
- Permits more face-to-face time for disease management

Adapted from Weiss P, Lowery K, Hess W. You've got E-mail: physician–patient electronic communication. Female Patient 2005;30:31–4.

Box 4
Disadvantages of e-mail communication

- Asynchronous communication
- Not appropriate for urgent/acute issues
- Privacy and confidentiality issues
- Not reimbursed by most insurers
- Potential for overuse by patients
- Cannot ensure that patient receives message

Adapted from Weiss P, Lowery K, Hess W. You've got E-mail: physician–patient electronic communication. Female Patient 2005;30:31–4.

---

to an example cited by Gunther Eysenbach, MD, in *The Impact of the Internet on Cancer Outcomes*, a "woman filed a lawsuit against a Radiologist, whose email address she found on a hospital Website and whom she asked a seemingly casual question via email. The Radiologist responded with a quick email trying to help. The woman later turned out to have cancer and claimed to have been harmed by the advice she received, and she sued the Radiologist."[23]

With the advent of social media, it is evident that the OB/Gyn can be vulnerable to more frequent legal contests by their patients. Although most patients gather information from the Internet to augment the facts and details their doctor is providing them, they also may be using social media and the Internet to follow-up on their physician's recommendations and treatment advice.[20] If the information the patient has researched on the Internet does not reflect what their OB/Gyn is recommending, it can pose legal problems or at the very least uncomfortable situations for the provider. Knowing this, the OB/Gyn should have a clear conversation with their newly diagnosed patient about using the information on the Internet and social media. The conversation should note that the Internet can contain accurate information but often also can expose them to misinformation that can do more harm than good. The OB/Gyn should discuss which web sites to browse, emphasizing those that are peer reviewed and nationally/internationally recognized. The patient should understand that there are individuals who post information online whose intent may not always be genuine and good.[24]

It is important for a physician to understand that it is human nature for a person facing a cancer diagnosis to seek out as much information as possible from as many sources as possible. A physician who understands this can be proactive and take measures to mitigate the legal risks and improve the doctor-patient relationship. As Farris Timimi states, the "opportunity as health care providers to partner with (our) patients has never been greater, yet all too often we allow risk averse fears to limit our ability to truly leverage our good content effectively to the online community. This risk adverse behavior truly limits our capacity to effectively engage our patients where they are – online."[25]

CREATE A STRONG PATIENT-DOCTOR RELATIONSHIP

It is impossible to diagnose breast cancers with 100% accuracy. Mammography, although currently the best tool for diagnosing breast cancer, is not 100% effective. Studies show that mammography will miss 10 to 30% of breast cancers.[10] By working together, breast imaging radiologists and OB/Gyns can help improve patient outcomes and reduce liability.

Physician Practice Question 4

Q: *How do OB/Gyns and radiologists work together to improve patient outcomes and reduce liability?*

A: *Increase patient satisfaction; listen to SBP self-reported symptoms; and create shared checklists*

Another way for a physician to reduce his or her liability is to increase patient satisfaction. Studies show a direct link to litigation and patient satisfaction. According to The Doctor's Company, a medical malpractice company, most breast cancer claims are filed because (1) the patient tells her doctor that she has found a lump and/or other symptom in her breast, and the appropriate appointments are not made in a timely fashion; (2) delay in diagnosis leads to a poor outcome for the patient; (3) the differences between screening and diagnostic mammography are not understood, so the incorrect test is ordered, resulting in delay of diagnosis; and (4) patient awareness and educational resources have increased, as have the patient's individual expectations.[26]

For years, studies have been conducted on the relationship between physician communication and malpractice suits. According to those studies, patients' perception of how much the physician cares can ultimately determine if the patient will bring a malpractice suit. In the event of a bad medical outcome, the patients' perception of the physician was one of the determining factors for pursing or not pursing a malpractice claim.[27] The communication style used directly impacts how the patient perceives the physician and will also impact their decision to pursue litigation.

One of the most basic communication techniques is listening. Patients know their bodies and need to be heard, but if the communication style involves a battery of questions, the physician may not hear what is really wrong with the patient. This encouragement of two-way conversation is often referred to as the "partnership model."[28] This model helps to promote patient participation, allows them to understand the appropriate medical options, and ensures they are accountable for their choices. This "shared decision-making" outlines treatment options for patients. The physician and patient agree on the course of treatment after discussing the advantages and disadvantages of each medical treatment.[29]

Developing this partnership with patients will encourage consistent, medically based approaches to patient populations and increases overall patient satisfaction. In addition, creating a final checklist of steps that can be reviewed with the patient helps to show consistency in care. By having this documented standard approach for all symptomatic breast patients, liability can be reduced and consistency in delivered care can be shown.

When creating the final checklist, focus should be placed on the SBP and the self-reported symptoms, as referenced previously in this article. All symptoms should be taken into account. Patient concerns will often be minimized and appropriate follow-up examinations will not be ordered.[28] Discounting of symptoms such as pain and/or patient age can prove detrimental to the patient outcome. Although these 2 indicators are not standard for a breast cancer presentation, these symptoms can be associated with malignancy.[29] The proven value of checklist documentation for CBE has been described previously by the authors and is recommended. In addition, a final checklist can be considered to reduce the likelihood of "perceived neglect" by the patient.[28] A sample of this checklist follows.

Final checklist: SBP with self-identified symptoms

A. Talk with the patient
B. Perform CBE and document findings on the CBE documentation form
C. Educate patient using the developed, standardized information regarding breast health and the value of mammography, in addition to high-risk evaluation
D. Refer the patient for a diagnostic mammogram and/or ultrasound, based on evidence-based guidelines. For example, the NCCN guidelines provide detailed recommendations and diagnostic algorithms for breast screening and diagnosis. Furthermore, it offers guidance for patient management, based on the clinical finding: palpable mass, nipple discharge, asymmetric thickening/nodularity, and skin changes (including inflammatory and Paget's disease).[30]
E. If SBP has positive diagnostic mammogram
   1. It is critical to follow evidence-based practice for SBP follow-up. The NCCN guidelines outline a detailed approach to management of patients with clinical symptoms, which includes patient follow-up based on BI-RADS categories. For BI-RADS categories 4 and 5, core biopsy is recommended and is the most common type of breast biopsy for tissue diagnosis. Radiologists in breast centers will also manage patients based on ACR recommendations for diagnostic mammography and/or ultrasound evaluation. Although NCCN indicates fine-needle aspiration as valuable in some clinical symptoms thought to be benign, it notes that cytologic experience is required in its pathology evaluation.[31]
   2. Work directly with the breast center facility staff, such as Breast Nurse Specialist, patient navigator, scheduler, technologist, and/or radiologist, to set up a biopsy and/or surgical referrals.
   3. Document the referral for the biopsy and the surgeon
F. If SBP has negative diagnostic mammogram
   1. Schedule a follow-up examination with the patient to discuss the desire for a surgical referral. Schedule the referral if the patient desires.
   2. If the patient chooses to follow the area of concern, document this and schedule a second follow-up appointment in 3 to 6 months. Do this before the patient leaves the office.
   3. If the patient does not keep the scheduled follow-up, communicate with the patient via either phone or letter and document the contact.

SELECTING A QUALITY BREAST CARE REFERRAL FACILITY

Selecting a quality breast referral facility and radiologist is a step all OB/Gyns should take with care–and they have choices in facilities and radiologists. Together, the OB/Gyn and breast referral facility and radiologists can work together on shared checklists for CBE, breast health education, high-risk evaluation, screening recommendations, and procedures when SBP present at either OB/Gyn practice or breast referral facility. A basic requirement for breast imaging facilities is confirming the facility's current accreditation by the ACR and Mammography Quality Standards Act (MQSA). Expanding the MQSA audit by adding additional quality performance measures demonstrates a breast referral facility's continued focus on the quality improvement and effectiveness of screening.[32,33]

The OB/Gyn must determine whether the facility's radiologist detects small, invasive breast cancer at the earliest stage, when survival is greatest. The volume of screening mammograms interpreted is an important indicator for radiologist performance and a minimum threshold in the United States is 480 per year based on MQSA requirements; yet this annual requirement is far smaller than in other countries.[31] Literature suggests that higher mammography volume does lead to improved performance.[32] It is recommended that the OB/Gyn seek facilities and radiologists who know and report additional quality metrics beyond volume alone, such as:

- Positive predictive value based on abnormal screen (5%–10%) and based on biopsy results (25%–40%); tumors found stage 0 or I (>50%)
- Minimal cancers found (>30%); cancers found per 1000 cases (screened-cancer detection rate) (2–10)
- Prevalent cancers found per 1000 first-time examinations (6–10)
- Incident cancers found per 1000 follow-up examinations (2–4).[32,33]

Consideration should be given to service levels to expedite care and reduce the patient's days-waiting for screening and diagnostic examinations, biopsy procedures, wire localizations, and ultimately surgical and oncologic interventions.

SUMMARY

OB/Gyns and radiologists should coordinate the care of their patients with breast disease through evidence-based practice and create shared processes and checklists. Shared processes and checklists, when predicated on evidence-based practice, creates standardization in diagnoses and appropriate follow- up of women with breast disease. Women with self-reported breast symptoms can be vulnerable to lack of-suitable follow-up, especially when OB/Gyns and radiologists do not have established checklists for managing their care. In this article, the authors have suggested tools for developing checklists for both SBP and ABP, in addition to how to assess the quality of OB/Gyn's selected imaging referral facility. Indeed, OB/Gyns and radiologists have an opportunity to share in the development of breast education for patients, including implementing the recommended components of ACOG's well-woman visit, evidence-based guidelines for breast cancer risk assessment (discussed in the article by Green elsewhere in this issue) sharing the reported statistics regarding screening mammography with patients. These strategies are designed not only to improve clinical outcome and satisfaction for patients but also to offer steps to help safeguard against litigation as well.

ACKNOWLEDGMENTS

The authors would like to thank Marjorie Gowdy and Claudia Z. Lee for their thoughtful comments and editing on this article.

REFERENCES

1. Whang J, Baker S, Patel R, et al. The causes of medical malpractice suits against radiologists in the United States [published online ahead of print November 30, 2012]. Radiology 2012. Available at: http://radiology.rsna.org/content/early/2012/11/28/radiol.12111119.full. Accessed December 6, 2012.
2. Berlin L, Berlin JW. Malpractice and radiologists in Cook County, IL: trends in 20 years of litigation. AJR Am J Roentgenol 1995;165(4):781.
3. American Congress of Obstetricians and Gynecologists. Medical Liability Climate Hurts Patients and Ob-Gyns. 2012. Available at: http://www.acog.org. Accessed December 6, 2012.
4. American Congress of Obstetricians and Gynecologists. 2011 Women's Health Statistics and Facts. 2012. Available at: http://www.acog.org/. Accessed December 6, 2012.

5. McGlynn EA, Asch SM, Adams J, et al. The quality of health care delivered to adults in the United States. N Engl J Med 2003;348(26):2635–45.
6. The Center for Health Affairs. The Emerging Field of Patient Navigation: A Golden Opportunity to Improve Healthcare. 2012. Available at: www.chanet.org. Accessed January 2, 2013.
7. American Cancer Society. Cancer treatment & survivorship facts & figures. Atlanta (GA): National Home Office: American Cancer Society Inc.; 2012. Available at: http://www.cancer.org/acs/groups/content/@epidemiologysurveilance/documents/document/acspc-033876.pdf. Accessed January 31, 2013.
8. Emanuel E, Tanden N, Altman S, et al. Sounding Board – A Systemic Approach to Containing Health Care Spending. N Engl J Med 2012;367(10):949–52.
9. Committee on Patient Safety and Quality Improvement. Committee opinion number 526: standardization of practice to improve outcomes. The American Congress of Obstetricians and Gynecologists; 2012. Available at: http://www.acog.org. Accessed December 6, 2012.
10. Brem RF, Baum J, Lechner M, et al. Improvement in sensitivity of screening mammography with computer-aided detection: a multiinstitutional trial. AJR Am J Roentgenol 2003;181(3):687–93.
11. American College of Radiology. Practice Guidelines for the Performance of Screening and Diagnostic Mammography. 2008. Available at: http://www.acr.org/~/media/ACR/Documents/PGTS/guidelines/Screening_Mammography.pdf. Accessed December 6, 2012.
12. California Department of Public Health Cancer Detection Section, Breast Expert Workgroup. Breast Cancer Diagnostic Algorithms for Primary Care Providers. 2011. Available at: http://www.qap.sdsu.edu. Accessed December 16, 2012.
13. Centers for Medicare and Medicaid Services (CMS). State Operations Manual Appendix A – Survey Protocol, Regulations and Interpretive Guidelines for Hospitals. Available at: http://www.cms.gov/regulations-and-guidance/guidance/manuals/downloads/som107ap_a_hospitals.pdf. Accessed December 18, 2012.
14. Duszak R, Berlin L. Malpractice issues in radiology: medicare compliance versus standard of care conformance – real or imaginary conflict? AJR Am J Roentgenol 2010;194:1552–8.
15. Kosters J, Gotzsche P. Regular self-examination or clinical examination for early detection of breast cancer. Cochrane Database Syst Rev 2002;(3):CD003373.
16. Committee on Gynecologic Practice. Committee opinion number 526: well-woman visit. The American College of Obstetricians and Gynecologists; 2012. Available at: http://www.acog.org. Accessed December 6, 2012.
17. United States Department of Health and Human Services: Agency for Healthcare Research and Quality. Guideline Summary NGC-8655, Breast Cancer Screening. Available at: http://www.guideline.gov/content.aspx?id=34275. Accessed January 2, 2013.
18. National Cancer Institute: Breast Cancer Surveillance Consortium. Reported as of December 27, 2009, NCI-funded Breast Cancer Surveillance Consortium co-operative agreement (U01CA63740, U01CA86076, U01CA86082, U01CA63736, U01CA70013, U01CA69976, U01CA63731, U01CA70040). Available at: http://breastscreening.cancer.gov/data/benchmarks/screening/2009/tableSensSpec.html. Accessed January 6, 2013.
19. Ziebland S, Chapple A, Dumelow C, et al. How the internet affects patients' experience of cancer: a qualitative study. BMJ 2004;328:564. Available at: http://dx.doi.org/10.1136/bmj.328.7439.564. Accessed January 15, 2013.

20. Lancellotti-Young C, Suk D. Internet and social change. Public policy 126s: Professor Rogerson. Available at: http://people.duke.edu. Accessed January 15, 2013.
21. The Canadian Medical Protective Association. Using email communication with your patient: legal risks. 2005. Available at: http://www.cmpa-acpm.ca. Accessed January 15, 2013.
22. Weiss P, Lowery K, Hess W. You've got E-mail: physician–patient electronic communication. Female Patient 2005;30:31–4.
23. Eysenback G. The impact of the Internet on cancer outcomes. CA Cancer J Clin 2003;53(6):356–71.
24. The Doctor-Patient Relationship in the Internet Age. Triple Helix Online. 2011. Available at: http://triplehelixblog.com/2011/09/the-doctor-patient-relationship-in-the-internet-age/. Accessed January 15, 2013.
25. Timimi F. Medicine, morality and health care social media. BMC Med 2012;10:83. Available at: http://www.biomedcentral.com/1741-7015/10/83. Accessed January 15, 2013.
26. Anderson RE. Breast Cancer: a Claims/Risk-Reduction Workshop. The Doctors Company. Available at: http://www.thedoctors.com/KnowledgeCenter/Patient Safety/articles/CON_ID_000298. Accessed January 11, 2013.
27. Strunk AL, Kenyon S. Medicolegal Considerations in the Diagnosis of Breast Cancer. Obstet Gynecol Clin North Am 2002;29(1):43–9.
28. Committee on Health Care for Underserved Women, Committee on Patient Safety and Quality Improvement. Committee opinion number 492: Effective patient-physician communication. The American College of Obstetricians and Gynecologists; 2011. Available at: http://www.acog.org. Accessed January 14, 2013.
29. Illinois State Medical Society. Limiting your liability in Breast/Cervical cancer and Pregnancy, vol. 8. Illinois Medicine EXPRESS; 2007 (4). Available at: http://www.isms.org/publications/imex/Pages/2007/04/2007_04e.aspx. Accessed January 11, 2013.
30. National Comprehensive Cancer Network (NCCN). Breast Cancer Screening and Diagnosis. 2013. Available at: NCCN.org. Accessed April 18, 2013.
31. Esserman L, Cowley H, Eberle C, et al. Improving the accuracy of mammography: volume and outcome relationships. J Natl Cancer Inst 2002;94(5):369–75.
32. Linver M. The expanded mammography audit: its value in measuring and improving your performance. Semin Breast Dis 2005;8(1):35–42.
33. Linver M, Osuch J, Brenner R, et al. Review article: the mammography audit: a primer for mammography quality standards act. AJR Am J Roentgenol 1995; 165:19–25.

Index

Note: Page numbers of article titles are in **boldface** type.

Obstet Gynecol Clin N Am 40 (2013) 599–609
http://dx.doi.org/10.1016/S0889-8545(13)00066-1
0889-8545/13/$ – see front matter © 2013 Elsevier Inc. All rights reserved.

Moving?

Make sure your subscription moves with you!

To notify us of your new address, find your **Clinics Account Number** (located on your mailing label above your name), and contact customer service at:

Email: **journalscustomerservice-usa@elsevier.com**

800-654-2452 (subscribers in the U.S. & Canada)
314-447-8871 (subscribers outside of the U.S. & Canada)

Fax number: **314-447-8029**

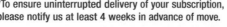

Elsevier Health Sciences Division
Subscription Customer Service
3251 Riverport Lane
Maryland Heights, MO 63043

*To ensure uninterrupted delivery of your subscription, please notify us at least 4 weeks in advance of move.

Printed and bound by CPI Group (UK) Ltd, Croydon, CR0 4YY

21/10/2024

01777179-0001